DISABILITY

THE BASICS

Disability: The Basics is an engaging and accessible introduction to disability which explores the broad historical, social, environmental, economic and legal factors which affect the experiences of those living with an impairment or illness in contemporary society. The book explores key introductory topics including:

- the diversity of the disability experience;
- disability rights and advocacy;
- ways in which disabled people have been treated throughout history and in different parts of the world;
- the daily realities of living with an impairment or illness;
- health, education, employment and other services that exist to support and include disabled people;
- ethical issues at the beginning and end of life.

Disability: The Basics aims to provide readers with an understanding of the lived experiences of disabled people and highlight the continuing gaps and barriers in social responses to the challenge of disability. This book is suitable for lay people, students of disability studies as well as students taking a disability module as part of a wider course within social work, health care, sociology, nursing, policy and media studies.

Tom Shakespeare is professor of disability research at Norwich Medical School, University of East Anglia. A sociologist by training, he has also contributed to debates in bioethics and cultural representation. He currently teaches medical students, social work students and others about working with disabled people. He researches independent living, mental health recovery and rehabilitation. He has been involved in the disability rights movement since 1986.

THE BASICS

For a full list of titles in this series, please visit www.routledge.com/The-Basics/book-series/B

DISABILITY

THE BASICS

Tom Shakespeare

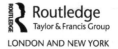

Routledge
Taylor & Francis Group

LONDON AND NEW YORK

First published 2018
by Routledge
2 Park Square, Milton Park, Abingdon, Oxon OX14 4RN

and by Routledge
711 Third Avenue, New York, NY 10017

Routledge is an imprint of the Taylor & Francis Group, an informa business

British Library Cataloguing-in-Publication Data
A catalogue record for this book is available from the British Library

Library of Congress Cataloging in Publication Data
Names: Shakespeare, Tom, 1966- author.
Title: Disability : the basics / Tom Shakespeare.
Description: Abingdon, Oxon ; New York, NY : Routledge, 2018. | Includes
bibliographical references and index.
Identifiers: LCCN 2017011075 | ISBN 978-1-138-65138-8 (hardback) |
ISBN 978-1-138-65139-5 (pbk.) | ISBN 978-1-315-62483-9 (ebook)
Subjects: LCSH: People with disabilities—Social conditions. | People with
disabilities—Great Britain—Social conditions. | Sociology of disabilities.
Classification: LCC HV1568 .S435 2018 | DDC 362.4—dc23
LC record available at https://lccn.loc.gov/2017011075

ISBN: 978-1-138-65138-8 (hbk)
ISBN: 978-1-138-65139-5 (pbk)
ISBN: 978-1-315-62483-9 (ebk)

Typeset in Bembo and Scala Sans
by FiSH Books Ltd, Enfield

Dedicated to Bill and Gill Albert

CONTENTS

PREFACE

The German critic and philosopher Walter Benjamin said once that the only reason to write a book yourself was because no one had written the book you wanted to read. That's my excuse for writing yet another book with the word 'disability' in the title. I have not come across a short basic book that enables the lay person, or the student, or the professional, to quickly grasp all the most important things about disability. That's what I am trying to do here, liberated from the need to provide references (although always based on the best contemporary evidence I can find). It's a political book, because I am committed in my research and practice to trying to improve the lives of disabled people. But while the style is conversational, I've also tried to be balanced and academically rigorous (if you want something more polemical, look at another introductory book by Roddy Slorach in the list of further reading at the end of Chapter 1).

I started postgraduate research in 1990 because I wanted to write a popular book about disability. Four years later, I still had not written the book, but I did have a doctorate. From there, my whole academic career began. In writing an accessible introduction now, I hope I am finally putting that initial motivation to rest. I am also drawing on other books that I have written over the years. I have not covered all the relevant issues here, partly because I am ignorant about many things, but also because of lack of space. But I hope I will give readers a good overview.

Chapter 1 gives an orientation in disability. I discuss definitions, terminology, disability prevalence, and explain something about the population. I also introduce the disability movement, who have been the major players in transforming understandings of disability. Chapter 2 tries to broaden the perspective, to look at how disability has been experienced in different places and at different times: I touch on historical moments such as the freak show, the workhouse, eugenics and institutions, and tell the stories of some notable individuals with impairments who made significant impacts on history. Chapter 3 looks at the life course of people with disabilities – children, working age people and older people – and tries to explore personal experiences such as independent living, but also risk of violence and abuse. In Chapter 4, I turn to look at disabling barriers in more detail, focusing on the physical and information environment, the role of negative attitudes, and the difficulties of achieving equal opportunities in employment. Chapter 5 discusses healthcare. Although it would be wrong simply to see disability as a health issue, disabled people have health needs and face barriers in getting those needs met. The chapter discusses prevention, access to mainstream health and rehabilitation, and then the specialist provision for people with learning difficulties and people with mental health conditions. In Chapter 6, I discuss education, including the debate between mainstream and special schools, and the difficulties disabled children face, in many parts of the developing world, in getting access to education at all. Chapter 7 turns to bioethics, and focuses on the issue of prenatal screening and assisted suicide, which have been very controversial among disability activists. Finally, Chapter 8 looks at the disability movement in a bit more detail, including different minorities within the disability community, and the role of disability arts and disability studies. As an appendix, I reprint a dialogue which I wrote twenty years ago about prenatal diagnosis, and which is as relevant as ever, plus a glossary of the terminology used in the book.

ACKNOWLEDGEMENTS

This book draws on research I have conducted alongside Nick Watson, Michael Wright, Sue Thompson, Tom Porter, Andrea Stockl, Nora Groce, Maria Kett, Joseph Simbaya, Richard Bwalya, Anthony Mugeere, Julius Omona, Andrew State, Emily Nayariki, Joyce Olenja, most of which has been funded by the Economic and Social Research Council, and the support and assistance of all of whom I acknowledge. It also draws on work I have done with Alana Officer, Sashka Posarac and others at the World Health Organization and the World Bank, to all of whom many thanks also. I would like to thank Bill Albert and Nick Watson for reading and commenting on a first draft of this book, and for all their advice, challenge and support to me over many years. Needless to say, any errors or infelicities are down to me, not these good people. On a personal level, thank you to Alice Whieldon for her continuing love and support, and patience during working weekends. I would also like to thank Bill and Gill Albert for their care and hospitality, particularly since I have been living in Norwich, and so would my dog, Winston, to whom they are second owners. With respect and love, I am dedicating this book to them.

UNDERSTANDING DISABILITY

Disability may be considered a minority issue. After all, only about 15 per cent of the population – one in seven – is disabled. But there are at least a billion people with disability on the planet, plus all their relatives and friends. So, most lives are touched by disability in some way, and it's about time we understood it better. Disability is both extremely interesting and rather complicated. As a social experience, it's in a process of transition – for better and for worse. Above all, disability is an experience that can affect anyone. You may not be born with an impairment, but you might develop a disease or have an accident. Most commonly, you could become impaired in older age. So, it's a matter of self-interest for everyone to learn a bit more about disability. And, when they know more, many people become less frightened of one day becoming disabled themselves.

The lives of disabled people in the UK have radically transformed over the last fifty years. In the 1960s, disabled people often lived in residential institutions. They usually attended segregated schools. Many disabled people did not work. Most public transport and buildings were inaccessible to them. There has been radical change over this period, as society has shifted from a very medicalised understanding of disability, where disabled people were considered people with unfortunate problems, and the duty of non-disabled people was to be charitable towards these victims and invalids; towards an understanding of disability as an equal opportunities issue, where disabled people have human rights and can make demands of society, as well as making contributions to it.

This book aims to give you an overview of both the evidence and the arguments about disability, in an accessible way. This first chapter will orient you in the field, providing a little background and offering you a straightforward approach to understanding disability. This should be relevant to everyone, but particularly to people who are planning to enter a profession which supports disabled people – like medicine or social work or education or rehabilitation therapies or nursing. The book is based on the United Kingdom, but will also give international comparisons and examples from developing countries, to show how disability depends on the context.

WHAT'S IN A NAME?

Anxieties about disabled people often coalesce around the appeal, 'But what do we call you?' Nobody wants to give offence, and there is an implied fear that disabled people are very sensitive. Traditional disability words – like 'spastic' or 'Mongol' or 'retarded' or 'deaf and dumb' – are now rightly regarded as objectionable by anyone who takes a moment to think about it. But there's also the implication that any worries about the status and treatment of disabled people are just another aspect of 'political correctness'. I've never heard anyone use terms like 'vertically challenged' except in jest. When people talk about 'differently abled', it feels like a slightly misguided liberal attempt to say that everyone has things they are more or less good at. But these neologisms discredit an important debate about language. Terminology reflects ways of thinking. Approaches to disability have radically changed, and the labels people use about themselves are symbolic of this wider shift (Table 1.1).

To start with, the disability terminology debate is about seeing people as persons first, rather than focusing on their medical conditions. So, for example, rather than 'epileptics' one might say instead 'people with epilepsy' – and similarly, 'people with schizophrenia'. Instead of 'learning disabled people' one might

Table 1.1 Some unacceptable and acceptable terms

Not acceptable	Acceptable
Handicapped	Disabled people (UK)
Crippled	People with disabilities (International)
Invalid	Person with chronic illness
Retarded	Person with learning difficulties
Spastic	Person with cerebral palsy
Deaf and dumb	Deaf or hard of hearing person
Mad	Person with mental health condition
Crazy	Service user
Psycho	Person with schizophrenia

say 'people with learning disabilities', which is the term used in the NHS. For the same reason, outside the UK, 'people with disabilities' is the preferred term for our community, because it is people-first language.

Second, it is a good principle to call people by the names they themselves prefer. For example, in the UK, 'People with learning difficulties' is preferred by people directly affected, and so it will be the phrase I use in this book – although in other English-speaking countries, 'people with intellectual disabilities' is more common. Another example is 'Deaf people', the capital D signifying that I am talking about a minority group with their own culture based around sign language, not just a group of people who can't hear.

Third, these sorts of terms shift the emphasis to the ways that society treats us. For that reason, 'disabled people' is the preferred term in the UK, because people want to emphasise how they are 'disabled by society', whereas 'impairment' refers to the underlying health condition. Impairments refer to things like being blind or deaf or having a mobility limitation or a cognitive difference (in a more scholarly book, I might be strict and use the term 'impairment' for individual issues and 'disability' for social issues, but here I will use the term 'disability' to refer to any aspect of the phenomenon). So the query about terminology is a useful one, because it gets to the heart of the complexity of disability. In practice, different people prefer different words. I always try to respect individual preferences, and not get too hung up on one word over another. For example, I am happy saying 'disabled people' and also happy saying 'people with disabilities'.

But should there be a collective noun at all? The idea that everyone with some sort of physical or mental impairment can be categorised together at all is rather new in human history. Prior to the early 1900s, it would have been unusual to have thought of all these people with so many different experiences as having anything in common. A variety of words were used – 'feeble-minded', 'cripple', 'blind', 'deaf and dumb', 'lunatic', 'insane' – it's interesting to note that most of these terms would be considered insults today. Back in 1915, the word 'handicap' started to be used, mainly of children, and in Britain and America it was more and more commonly employed to connote people with a range of impairments. Around the same time, 'disability', which had previously signified legal restrictions, was transferred for use as a collective noun. As the disability rights movement became stronger, so the term 'handicap' became associated with out-dated approaches. A false etymology associated the word with begging, and by extension charity, to which the new disability activists were vigorously opposed. Increasingly, like 'homosexual' as a term for gay people, 'handicap' became an inappropriate term for referring to an individual or a group.

A collective noun is debatable partly because disability is very diverse. The body or mind can be damaged or limited or changed in many different ways. Some conditions are usually obvious at birth – for example cerebral palsy or Down syndrome. Some issues become evident when a child does not develop like other children – for example, autistic spectrum conditions. Then there are traumatic injuries such as head injury or spinal cord injury that strike out of the blue, often affecting active young men who take risks or work in dangerous occupations. Some adult illnesses are episodic or degenerative – like depression or multiple sclerosis. Finally, there are conditions mainly associated with ageing, such as stroke or dementia. As well as these differences of onset, it's also obvious that some impairments are visible – for example, restricted growth or phocomelia (a congenital condition causing limb defects, associated with use of the drug thalidomide in pregnancy) – and other conditions are invisible – like epilepsy or depression or heart disease.

This diversity of disability explains why it took centuries for 'disabled people' to be considered as having something in common, regardless of our differences. It's probably true to say that it took even longer for us to think of ourselves as one community. Why would someone with paraplegia think they had anything in common with someone who experiences mental illness? She might say to herself 'I may not be able to walk, but at least my mind is working normally'. When we conducted research with people with restricted growth, many of them insisted: 'I am different, not disabled'. A government research project in 2003 found that more than half of those who could be defined as disabled, do not think of themselves as disabled. Apart from the diversity of experiences, the main reason people do not want to be labelled as disabled, is because disability remains a stigmatised identity. Nobody wants to be categorised in a way which seems limiting or negative. They want to stress their similarity to others, not their differences; what they can do, not what they cannot do.

WHY GENERALISING ABOUT DISABILITY IS DANGEROUS

Disability is a multi-dimensional concept, which should be understood in terms of a continuum. Human perfection does not exist. Everyone is limited in some way, whether it's a minor blemish or an allergy or something more serious. But most people would not consider themselves disabled, even if they have an impairment. There are many types of disability, and it affects people in different ways and to a greater or lesser extent. Compare this with gender: there are a tiny number of intersex people, and a growing but still small number of trans people. The vast majority of people – more than 99 per cent of the human population – are either men or women. There are different ways of being masculine or feminine, but there are certain generalisations which apply across a culture. You can generalise about gender, up to a point (although you have to be very careful that you're not just reproducing cultural stereotypes).

Because disability is diverse, it can be tricky to characterise it. For example, we might point to the evidence that says disabled people usually report a good quality of life, in fact, sometimes disabled people report a quality of life that is better than non-disabled people. This counter-intuitive claim has been found true in many surveys. But then we have to acknowledge that this fact does not usually apply to disabled people who experience pain. Constant or extreme pain makes life very much more difficult, and undermines quality of life. We could argue strongly that disabled people can work, that employment barriers should be removed, and that disabled people can make a contribution in most sectors of the economy, whether or not they have a physical or mental impairment. Yet people with severe learning difficulties (also known as profound and multiple intellectual disability, PMID) will be unable to do a job, and people with severe forms of mental illness will also find it difficult to do regular work.

The tendency to make generalisations, with the best of intentions, can cause problems. If disability is on a continuum, and if people are generalising about disability on the basis of one end or the other end of the continuum, then they are likely to disagree with each other because they are talking about different phenomena. For example, in the debate around prenatal testing, discussed in Chapter 7, advocates of screening talk about the benefits of avoiding the births of disabled people who will lead restricted lives, full of suffering. Those who oppose selective abortion talk about the achievements which disabled people can attain in their lives. Both sides in this argument are correct. In some cases, disability has a very profound impact on individuals and on their families. But in other cases, disabled people succeed as well as, or better than, non-disabled people. Therefore the argument about screening becomes harder to resolve, because the two sides use the same term 'disability' to refer to different experiences.

This book is an attempt to describe the whole disability experience, albeit at a very basic level. I am trying to cover people with physical impairments, people with sensory impairments such as sight and hearing loss, people with learning difficulties, people with mental health conditions, and people with chronic illnesses. The latter group are often ignored. Their impairments – such as respiratory diseases, or heart disease, or rheumatism – may be invisible, even though they are among the commonest forms of disability. People with chronic illness often do not identify as disabled. Yet they are limited in their functioning and often their participation, and they are also vulnerable to disabling barriers. Another group often ignored are older people, who make up half of all disabled people. Often their impairments are just seen as a natural part of growing old.

HOW MANY PEOPLE ARE DISABLED?

The discussion of the category 'disability' should alert us to the difficulties of coming up with a reliable figure for the number of disabled people (the discussion here gets increasingly detailed and technical, so feel free to skip ahead to Table 1.2). For example, in 1969, the UK Office of Population, Census and Surveys (OPCS) conducted a survey which produced the estimate that there were 1,130,000 who were handicapped, and 1,942,000 who were impaired but not handicapped, a total of 3,071,000. In 1988, a second OPCS survey found that there were 5,780,000 adults in Great Britain with one or more disabilities. Why had the numbers nearly doubled in less than twenty years? The reason was the first survey referred to physical impairments which limited life, and emphasised ability for self-care. The second survey was more far-reaching, included all types of impairments and set a lower threshold.

Disability is a social category, so any prevalence estimate will depend on the definition of disability we adopt, and the boundaries of the category. You could go with a subjective definition – which would capture all the people who want to identify as disabled. But we have already discovered that many people who, objectively, we would define as having an impairment do not want to identify as disabled. There may also be some people whose disability status we may be sceptical about – like obese people – who might want the label for themselves. When it comes to entitlement for a blue disabled parking badge, many people would like to be counted as disabled. Is a person who is short-sighted disabled? Probably not, because almost everyone who has refractive error has spectacles that correct vision. But think of having a sight or hearing impairment in a country where you could not get glasses or a hearing aid, or batteries for a hearing aid. You would find it very hard to learn at school, and you would be disadvantaged in the job market.

When I worked at the World Health Organization (WHO), I was part of the team who wrote the first *World Report on Disability*, and one of our tasks was coming up with a new global prevalence estimate for disability. This number derived from the World Health Survey (WHS), using data from 59 countries, and tens of thousands of respondents. A module of the WHS asked questions about functioning in 8 areas of life (affect, cognition, relationships, mobility, pain, sleep and energy, self-care and vision). The answers were compiled onto a composite disability scale from 0 to 100. A threshold of 40 was chosen as the dividing line between 'disabled' and 'non-disabled', partly because people with commonly accepted disabilities (e.g. blindness, paraplegia) were scoring around 40. This produced an average prevalence figure, for adults, of 15.6 per cent who experienced significant difficulties in functioning. The number who experienced very significant difficulties was estimated as 2.2 per cent. This research found that poorer people, women and older people had higher rates of impairment and that the rate was higher in lower-income countries than in higher-income countries.

Although it had a different definition and approach to disability, we also took into account the figures obtained from the Global Burden of Disease (GBD) study in 2004 (19.4 per cent of adults and 5.1 per cent of children experiencing 'moderate or severe disability'). Combining the GBD and WHS figures, and extrapolating to include children, the WHO and the World Bank *World Report on Disability* suggested that, overall, 15 per cent of the world's population had significant disability, equivalent to one billion people.

Two things should be noted about this figure. First, it is higher than the 1970s WHO estimate of 10 per cent prevalence. But the 1970s figure always had a 'back of an envelope' feel to it. Second, the new estimate is much higher than the prevalence obtained from surveys conducted in low-income countries, which have tended to come up with a figure of 2–3 per cent. The reason for the latter is that household surveys generally entail asking people about a range of obvious impairments: blindness, deafness, mobility impairment, intellectual impairment. The majority of disabled people are not covered by these traditional categories. When I am teaching my students about disability, I always point out that the category is rather elastic, and that any measurement is an artefact – it derives from the questions we are asking.

Turning to the UK, I will try to give a snapshot of how many people are disabled, and what sort of impairments are most common. While 30 per cent of the population (15 million people in England) have a *long-term illness*, a lower proportion, 18 per cent, have a *limiting long-standing illness* (ONS 2012). These two terms derive from the UK Census and the British General Household Survey, and evidence shows that self-reporting of limiting long-standing illness depends not just on clinical situation, but also on social, environmental and psychological factors such as isolation. Increasingly, people have more than one condition: the number of people with three or more conditions is forecast to rise by a third by 2018. The WHO figure of 15 per cent of the population having a disabling impairment is close to this UK figure of 18 per cent of the population having a limiting long-standing illness.

Having established the magnitude of the issue, let's understand more about this group of people with impairments. It's important to note that there is an age gradient in disability prevalence. We might think of congenital conditions such as muscular dystrophy or dwarfism as typical, but in fact only around 2 per cent of births are affected by impairment. Approximately 5 per cent of children, 10 per cent of working-age adults and up to 50 per cent of older people have disabilities. As the population ages, the number of disabled people in the population will increase, although the percentage of older people who are disabled is not increasing. In 2009, it was predicted that there would be an 86 per cent rise in the number of disabled people aged 65 and above by 2026. Seventy-nine per cent of disabled people over state pension age reported that they acquired their impairment after the age of 50, and 47 per cent over the age of 65. Over two-thirds of people over the age of 85 are disabled.

As well as this association with age, there is also a socio-economic gradient, in other words you are more likely to be disabled if you are poor. Seven per cent of adults in higher mana-gerial, administrative and professional occupations are defined as disabled according to the Equality Act, compared with 12 per cent of adults in semi-routine occupations. Rates of disability are higher in the north of England and in Wales than in the south of England, and are higher in poorer local authority areas (35 per cent in Port Talbot or Blaenau Gwent versus 15 per cent in City of London and 17 per cent in Wandsworth. Those in the bottom fifth of the income distribution face a risk of becoming disabled two and a half times as high as those in the top fifth of the distribution.

Women are more likely to report health problems than men, with 63 per cent of men reporting the absence of health problems, compared with 55 per cent of women, according to the England Health Survey 2012. In terms of ethnicity, around a third of Pakistani or Bangladeshi people in UK are covered by the disability provisions of the Equality Act, compared with around a quarter of white, Indian and black British people. Children with special educational needs (SEN) consequent on learning disabilities are more likely to be male and from poorer families. Moderate and severe learning difficulties are more common among children from Traveller and Roma communities. Profound multiple learning difficulties are more common among children of Pakistani or Bangladeshi descent.

The major causes of disability are musculo-skeletal, particularly arthritis and rheumatism, accounting for about 30 per cent of all disability across Europe. In terms of years lived with disability, depression ranks third in UK and second globally. Overall, 18 per cent of working-age adults have a Common Mental Disorder. Just under a fifth (18 percent) of all adults experience long-term pain, 13 percent have chronic health conditions and 8 percent have a mobility impairment. Sight loss affects about two million people in the UK, including an estimated 80,000 of working age and 25,000 children. The prevalence of visual impairment is higher among those with multiple disability and older people. Twenty per cent of people aged over 75, and 50 per cent of those over age 90 years in the UK are living with sight loss, while 55 per cent of people over 60 and 90 per cent of patients over 81 have a hearing loss. In England in 2010, it was estimated that 1,198,000 people had learning disabilities, or just over 2 per cent of the population. While conditions like Down syndrome, Fragile X and autism are common diagnoses in learning disabilities, the majority of learning disability is of unknown origin.

Once again, it's important to note that data on disability are complex and contested. So the table below is a best estimate. Research and data collection use varying definitions and thresholds, and these have changed over time. Studies obtain different results depending on whether they rely on self-report or clinical diagnosis of health conditions associated with disability, and whether they ask about specific health conditions, or measure general functioning. Currently, there are efforts to standardise data collection, to promote use of the International Classification of Functioning, Disability and Health (ICF), and thus to achieve comparability of national and international disability data.

THE BEGINNINGS OF DISABILITY POLITICS

Now we know what we're talking about, it is time to turn to the question of why we are talking about it. In other words, how did disability become a political issue, and when did we begin re-thinking our basic assumptions about disability? Although there had been mass demonstrations as early as the 1930s, the first stirrings of the contemporary disabled people's movement began in the 1960s. Many different campaigns were starting in this period,

Table 1.2 UK disability prevalence figures

Condition	Number of people affected
People with a long-term illness	19 million
People affected by common mental disorders	11 million
People affected by pain	11 million
Disabled people	10 million
People with hearing loss	9 million
Unpaid carers	6 million
People with sight loss	2 million
People with learning difficulties	1.28 million
People with dementia	850,000
People with autism	640,000
People with spinal cord injury	40,000
First language sign language users	17,000
People with restricted growth	6,000

Note: 2016 estimates based on UK population 64.1 million.

such as the Child Poverty Action Group (founded in 1965) and Shelter, the homelessness and housing organisation (founded in 1966). Flaws in the post-war welfare state were becoming evident to a population which was becoming more educated. People were seeing the problems in their own lives, realising that these were social issues, not private woes, meeting in groups to discuss them, and becoming activists to protest against them. The disability movement followed the same trajectory of previous movements: the Civil Rights movement in America was followed by the women's movement, and then the lesbian and gay liberation movement, and finally the disabled people's movement. This pattern occurred in USA, in UK, and in many other developed countries, and during the 1980s and 1990s in developing countries as well.

Like most social movements, the disability movement comprised a range of voices and perspectives. Organisations run by non-disabled people were active, alongside organisations of disabled people and of carers of disabled people. In the late 1960s, the UK campaign focused on welfare benefits, particularly benefits for married disabled women who had never worked. Demonstrations were held and social policy research was conducted – all in a rather decorous way. But some groups of disabled people argued strongly that the political agenda should be much broader, and adopted more strident tones. One of these groups was the Union of the Physically Impaired Against Segregation (UPIAS). UPIAS had formed after Paul Hunt, a resident in the Le Court Cheshire home in Hampshire, wrote a letter to *The Guardian* newspaper, calling for the formation of a user group of people living in residential care. He later joined with Vic Finkelstein, a paralysed South African psychologist who had been expelled for his anti-apartheid activities and come to Britain. UPIAS was a small, Marxist-inspired group of disabled people, who spent time thinking through the disability problem.

The analysis they came up with became known as the 'social model' of disability, after the disabled sociologist Michael Oliver began to publish academic articles about it in the 1980s. But the kernel of the idea came in 1976 in a small UPIAS booklet called *Fundamental Principles*:

> In our view, it is society which disables physically impaired people. Disability is something imposed on top of our impairments, by the way we are unnecessarily isolated and excluded from full participation in society.

In other words, the emphasis of the radical disability movement switched from individual problems, to the wider oppression and social barriers that excluded and disabled people. UPIAS felt it was not enough to campaign for benefits, as the Disablement Income Group had been doing for the last decade. The disability problem was deeper and more complex. For that reason, 'disabled people' became the preferred term that activists used, highlighting that people were disabled by society, not by their bodies. Using the term 'disabled people', rather than 'people with disabilities', became a marker for the radical wing of the disability community.

This redefinition of disability from 'medical model' to 'social model' in the British disability movement parallels the women movement's redefinition of women's experience in the early 1970s. Feminists like Anne Oakley and others had distinguished between *sex* – the biological difference between male and female – and *gender*, the socio-cultural distinction between men and women, or masculine and feminine. The former was biological and universal, the latter was social, and specific to particular times and places. Thus it could be claimed that sex corresponds to impairment, and gender corresponds to disability. *Impairment* is the deficit of body or mind; *disability* is the social oppression and exclusion. The disability movement was following the well-established political path of de-naturalising forms of social oppression, demonstrating that what was believed to be biological and unchanging was actually a product of specific ways of thinking and responding to people with impairments.

For example, Vic Finkelstein wrote a famous article about a village, which was well-adapted to people who used wheelchairs. Everything was level, surfaces were at the right height, bathrooms were spacious. But then some walking people came to live in the village, and started complaining that they kept on hitting their heads, and that their backs ached from bending down to the lower level counters. The point of the parable was to show that it was social arrangements, not forms of embodiment, which constituted the problem – and that they could be altered.

A NEW SOCIAL MOVEMENT

In Britain, the fledgling disabled people's movement coalesced around the British Council of Organisations of Disabled People, founded in 1981. This federation comprised all the local and national organisations 'of' disabled people, as opposed to the traditional charitable organisations like Leonard Cheshire, Scope (then the Spastics Society), RNIB and RNID who were all 'for' disabled people. A key principle of the disabled people's movement, throughout the world, has been the principle of self-organisation, following the slogan 'nothing about us without us'. Disabled Peoples' International was also founded in 1981, splitting away from Rehabilitation International, the traditional global federation of disability organisations. In each case, the majority of the groups affiliating to these new peak bodies were cross-impairment organisations. Typically, each city or region of the UK would have a coalition of disability organisations which each represented different health conditions or interests – for example, mental health groups, Deaf people's groups, groups of people with learning difficulties, local independent living groups and so on. So for example, there was Avon Coalition of Disabled People, or Greater Manchester Coalition of Disabled People, or Lothian Coalition of Disabled People.

The British social model has been called 'the big idea' of the disability movement, and it has been globally influential. This big idea has had two major impacts. First, it identified a political strategy: barrier removal. If people with impairments are disabled by society, then the priority is to dismantle these disabling barriers, in order to promote the inclusion of people with impairments. Rather than pursuing a strategy of cure or rehabilitation, it would be better to pursue a strategy of social transformation. In particular, if disability could be proven to be the result of discrimination, then campaigners for anti-discrimination legislation regarded civil rights – on the model of the Americans with Disabilities Act, and the British Equal Opportunities and Race Relations laws – as the ultimate solution.

The second impact of the social model was on disabled people themselves. Replacing a traditional 'deficit' approach with a social oppression understanding was, and remains, very liberating for disabled individuals. Suddenly, people realised that it was society that was at fault, not themselves. They didn't need to change; society needed to change. They didn't have to be sorry for themselves; rather, they could be angry. The social model was transformative on individuals and built a strong political identity. Just as with feminist 'consciousness-raising' in the seventies, or with lesbians and gays 'coming out', so disability activists began to think of themselves in a totally new way. They become empowered to mobilise for equal citizenship and independent living. Rather than a demeaning reliance on charity, disabled activists could now demand their rights. The disability movement became another example of identity politics, alongside the women's movement, gay liberation and the movements of black and ethnic minority people.

For researchers, the social model opened up new lines of enquiry. Whereas medical sociologists had traditionally investigated issues such as individual adjustment to impairment, the social model inspired researchers in the new field of disability studies to turn their attention to topics such as discrimination, the relationship between disability and industrial capitalism, or the varying cultural representations of people with impairment. The social model enabled the focus to be widened from studying individuals to exposing broader social and cultural processes. Disability studies self-consciously emulated the precedents of Marxism, feminism, lesbian and gay studies and post-colonial studies, all of which intellectual currents had prompted new questions and generated new insights and evidence on the basis of an overt political affiliation with social movements of liberation.

FROM BARRIERS TO INCLUSION TO HUMAN RIGHTS

UPIAS and other disability activists of the 1970s were fighting to escape from residential institutions and live in the community. The principle of independent living was about saying that disabled people had all the same needs as everyone else – for information, health, housing, transport and so on – but that those normal needs were not ordinarily met. The reason for failure to meet these ordinary needs was social barriers.

So what were the barriers that made life more difficult for disabled people? The original policy statement of UPIAS set out an agenda:

> We find ourselves isolated and excluded by such things as flights of steps, inadequate public and personal transport, unsuitable housing, rigid work routines in factories and offices, and a lack of up-to-date aids and equipment.
>
> (UPIAS Aims paragraph 1)

This list of mainly physical barriers reflected the fact that most UPIAS members were wheelchair users. The concept of disabling barriers and enabling environments has since been expanded to show that simple changes can make life easier for people with sight or hearing loss; that assistive devices and clearer text can help people with dyslexia; that flexible working can help people with mental health conditions. The legal concept of 'reasonable adjustment' refers to these various accommodations which equalise the environment for disabled people and promote inclusion.

But barriers are more than just environmental. Discrimination in education or employment or healthcare, as this book will argue, also render disabled people second class citizens. It is often easier to fit a ramp or provide screen reader software than to change the prejudices which are so often associated with disability. For example, there is considerable stigma surrounding mental illness. People think that those who have experienced bipolar disorder or schizophrenia are unreliable or dangerous. Partly as a result, people with mental illness suffer worse health outcomes than other people; they are more likely to be unemployed; and they are more likely to be victims of violence. The 'Time to Change' campaign led by MIND and Rethink Mental Illness is about challenging the stigma associated with mental illness, and showing it is an ordinary part of life.

In summary, the main barriers – environmental and other – include the following:

- inaccessible public transport;
- inaccessible public buildings;
- signage, communication and information in inaccessible formats;
- negative attitudes;
- low expectations;
- prejudiced cultural representations;
- discrimination in healthcare;
- discrimination in employment; and
- violence and abuse.

The disability movement campaigned throughout the 1980s and 1990s for civil rights legislation and independent living. In 1990, Colin Barnes's book *Disabled People in Britain and Discrimination* documented that disabled people faced discrimination in many areas of life. In 1992, the mainstream disability charities joined the radical movement in one unified 'Rights Now' campaign which brought hundreds of thousands of disabled people onto the streets. Finally, the campaign bore fruit, when the Conservative government finally passed the 1995 Disability Discrimination Act. It became illegal to treat disabled people differently to non-disabled people, and employers had to provide reasonable adjustments for disabled employees and remove barriers to access. The subsequent Labour government strengthened provisions through the Disability Rights Commission Act 1999, and the Disability Discrimination Act of 2005. As well ensuring accessibility of public transport, the latter also created the disability equality duty, whereby all public bodies had to develop and report on strategies to promote equality. Finally, the 2010 Equality Act brought together legislation covering all forms of discrimination, although it also watered down enforcement of the duty on public bodies to promote disability equality which had been an important feature of the 2005 legislation.

At the global level, in 2006 the United Nations General Assembly agreed the Convention on the Rights of Persons with Disabilities (CRPD), a new treaty to promote, protect and ensure the human rights of the billion disabled people in the world. The CRPD came into force in May 2008, and by the time of writing, 172 countries have ratified it. This means that their domestic law should be interpreted and applied in the light of the rights that the CRPD outlines through its fifty articles. Those articles cover familiar issues like access and attitudes, transport, education, health and employment. The CRPD was the first human rights treaty of the twenty-first century, but it follows the same pattern as the Convention on the Rights of the Child, the Convention on the Ending of All Forms of Discrimination Against Women, the Convention Against Torture, and other global legal standards which seek to establish a fair and equal treatment for everyone in society.

Many of those who discuss the CRPD state that it does not create new human rights, it simply applies existing human rights to disabled people, who have for so long been denied them. I am not sure that's correct. In previous human rights treaties, it was not necessary, for example, to state that everyone has legal capacity, or that everyone has the right to live in the community. These things were taken for granted by non-disabled people, but have to be specified and defended for disabled people. The CRPD is also innovative in specifying what has to be done on a global scale, through international development cooperation, to ensure that disabled people in developing countries also have the chance of having their rights realised. The CRPD specifies both the traditional civil and political rights – for example, liberty and security and political participation – but also social and economic rights – for example education and employment. This again is innovative. Some of these rights are liberty rights, which outline freedoms for disabled people, and others are claim rights, which entail obligations on rights-bearers, such as nation states, for example to provide social protection.

If the CRPD were fully implemented, the barriers which exclude and disabled people would be removed and an equal playing field established, and disabled people would be able to achieve independent living. The ongoing work of the UN Committee on the Rights of Persons with Disabilities is to hold countries to account and to help them progressively realise the rights of disabled people. Every three years, each 'state party' to the CRPD has to report on what it has done to promote, protect and ensure the human rights of disabled people. The government submits the official report, and civil society submits one or more shadow reports, usually pointing out the problems. The Committee listens, questions the country representatives, and then makes recommendations, in the form of observations about how the situation should be improved. Most countries take these hearings, and the investigations carried out by the Committee, very seriously. However, and shamefully, when the UK government was investigated by the Committee, leading to their 2016 report on 'grave and systematic violations' of the human rights of disabled people, the relevant UK government minister called their approach 'patronising and offensive', and rejected their critique.

BEYOND DICHOTOMIES

For all its strengths, the social model is a crude approach to disability. It was never intended to be a social theory to explain everything. It sets up a dichotomy between the so-called medical model and the social model. On a crude interpretation, it risks implying that there is no place for medical or rehabilitation approaches to disability. By emphasising the structural aspects so strongly, it neglects the personal dimension of living with an impairment. This has made it harder for many disabled people to identify with the social model. In the 2009 British Social Attitudes Survey, a majority of respondents (47 per cent) believed that it was a combination of health problems, and attitudes and barriers in society, which limit disabled people. In fact, in this survey, disabled people were slightly more likely than non-disabled people to see their health problems as the cause of disadvantage. Other surveys have found similar things. The social model is not intuitive, even to disabled people themselves. It reduces a complex reality to a simplistic picture, which people with impairments or illnesses may find it difficult to identify with.

From the research I have conducted and read about, from the conversations I have had with other disabled people, and from my own life experience, I have come to the conclusion that disability is multi-factorial. In other words, it results from the interplay of many different factors.

At the individual level, there is the impairment itself, and its impact on functioning. Does it cause pain? Is it visible or invisible? Can it be treated? What does it stop you doing? Then there are the psychological consequences of having an impairment, together with the personality that a person has (are they optimistic or pessimistic, are they extroverted or introverted, and so on). Then what are the psychological or emotional consequences of the way that the individual is treated in society? What are the beliefs that the individual has about their potential and their expectations?

At the level of society, there are all the external factors: not just the physical environment (including the natural environment), but also the social environment. How are disabled people treated? How strong are family networks? What expectations does society have of them? Are reasonable adaptations provided? Are assistive technologies provided? Is there access to educational and employment opportunities? What are the cultural representations of this impairment or disability in general? What are the attitudes to disabled people with this impairment? Is this a society which strives for equal rights for disabled people?

These individual and societal – or intrinsic and extrinsic – factors combine to produce the unique experience of disability that a specific individual has in a particular place at a certain point in human history. As UPIAS argued, oppression makes everything worse. But disability is more than just oppression. For this reason, disability differs from the other identity politics issues referred to earlier. Thinking of people who are from a minority ethnic community, if you remove racism and discrimination from the equation, there is no reason why they cannot flourish and compete equally with the majority ethnic community. For women, unless they are made solely responsible for home-making and child-rearing, there is no intrinsic reason why they cannot do as well as men in almost every occupational setting and sector of society. Similarly for gay people. Yet for disabled people, even after discrimination and prejudice is removed, inequalities are likely to remain. The level playing field does not liberate everyone. For some people with impairments, barrier removal is enough. For others, particularly those with profound intellectual impairments, the individual free market economy is not a place where they will flourish. They cannot work in all the same roles, or at the same intensity. This caveat applies also to people with severe mental illness, who may find regular employment impossible. There is a requirement for extra support and protection in order that they can lead lives of an equal quality to other disabled and non-disabled people.

This book is based on this understanding that disability is multi-factorial. This echoes the account in the WHO International Classification of Functioning, Disability and Health, which talks about a bio-psycho-social model. In this approach, all the different factors should be given weight. We cannot reduce the complexity of disability to either a biological problem, a psychological problem, or a social problem. We need to take account of all the factors, and intervene at all the different levels to benefit and include disabled people. This means medical and rehabilitation interventions; assistive devices; psychological support; barrier removal; supportive welfare benefits; legal protections; cultural change. Different interventions will be appropriate for different people in different settings, within the overall context of the human rights agenda established by the CRPD.

This also has implications for prevention. In Chapter 7, we will look more closely at issues around bioethics, and in particular genetics. But it's important to state that the multi-factorial approach to disability also implies that prevention of health conditions leading to disability can be part of the response, so long as this is done in an ethical way. For example, there is currently a global effort to rid the world of poliomyelitis, a disabling viral infection that causes paralysis and sometimes death. The virus was first identified in 1908; in the US, the peak of the epidemic was 1952, when 21,000 cases of paralysis were reported; effective vaccines were introduced from 1955, and the numbers fell. Today, only a few countries still have endemic polio and the hope is to eradicate the disease completely. People affected by polio have achieved great things, from President Franklin D. Roosevelt to the singers Joni Mitchell and Ian Dury, or the disability activist Ed Roberts. Yet few people doubt that it is desirable to prevent more people contracting the disease. It's entirely possible to support and celebrate people affected by an illness or impairment, while still trying to prevent further people being affected by it. To take another example, the slogan of the QuadPara Association of South Africa, a disabled people's organisation, is: 'Drive carefully: we don't want new members!'

CONCLUSION

Although the response to disabled people in Britain has radically changed in the last fifty years, we have not achieved full realisation of human rights or social inclusion. Neither the UK disability discrimination legislation nor the global Convention on the Rights of Persons with Disabilities has equalised the situation of disabled people. Almost all UK public buildings and most public transport is now accessible to disabled people – the situation is even better in the USA. Yet less than half of British disabled people are in employment (46.3 per cent), according to 2012 figures, compared with more than three quarters of non-disabled people (76.4 per cent), an employment gap of 30 percentage points. In 2013, there were still 35,000 adults with learning difficulties living in some form of residential institutions in England. Between 2007 and 2015, the percentage of all children who were educated in segregated settings increased over this period from 1.1 to 1.2 per cent. This expansion of segregated education represents an increase from 90,350 to 104,355 children. All these details show that there is still a long way to go until full disability equality is realised in the UK. Britain is one of the richest countries in the world and has better provision than most developed countries, so disabled people in Britain are still better off than they are in the majority of the world.

As stated at the beginning of the chapter, disability affects everyone. This is because almost every extended family includes a person affected by disability. It's also because everyone is at risk of becoming disabled. Accidents or disease could happen to anyone, and everyone will age and acquire limitations or impairments. Disability is not a tragedy, but it's not just an irrelevant difference. I have argued that the best way of thinking about it is as a predicament, which many people have to face in life, and which everyone should think about. Good societies enable people to cope with this predicament by removing barriers, providing supports, and by treating disability as part of normal human variation, rather than an abnormality to be discarded. Everyone affects disability.

FURTHER READING

Jane Campbell and Michael Oliver. 1996. *Disability Politics: understanding our past, changing our future*. London: Routledge.

James Charlton. 1998. *Nothing About Us, Without Us: disability oppression and empowerment*. Berkeley, CA: University of California Press.

Roddy Slorach. 2016. *A Very Capitalist Condition: a history and politics of disability*. London: Bookmarks Publications.

World Health Organization and World Bank. 2011. *World Report on Disability*. Geneva: World Health Organization.

DISABILITY ACROSS TIME AND PLACE

Disability is not simply a natural phenomenon: it is always influenced by social relations and cultural values. Whereas illness and impairment have been experienced across human existence, there have been very different reactions to it, from incarceration, to elimination, to fascination and sometimes inclusion. In different societies, disabled people have lived very different lives. Just as impairment and disability are very variable, so also cultural reactions are similarly diverse. For example, blind people have been very respected in some cultures, but not in others. People with epilepsy have often been feared or stigmatised, because they are believed to be possessed by spirits. Disability in old age has been considered normal and inevitable, but older people have also often been venerated. Children with disabilities have sometimes been killed or left to die. Limitations of space mean that this chapter can only offer little more than a series of snapshots or moments in the history of disability, highlighting varying responses to impairment around the world at different times, together with some portraits of individual disabled people.

DISABILITY IN ANCIENT AND MEDIEVAL SOCIETIES

Only traces can be discovered about disability in times past. In many societies, disabled children would have been left to die, as famously happened in ancient Sparta, with its militarist ethos. The Greek philosopher Aristotle wrote, 'As to the exposure of children, let there be a law that no deformed child shall live.' The Romans, too, practised exposure of disabled children. Societies surviving on the edge of scarcity are not sentimental regarding children who may not be able to contribute economically. The anthropologist Mary Douglas writes of the Nuer people in Africa, who traditionally regarded disabled children as offspring of the hippopotamus, and so placed them in the river to drown. Still today, children with severe disabilities are left to die in parts of the developing world.

However, this approach was not ubiquitous in the ancient world: the Roman writer Strabo describes Egypt as 'the land where all children are reared', and exposure of disabled children was forbidden there. In particular, dwarfs were celebrated under the Pharaohs. There was even a dwarf Bes, who was the god of love, sexuality and childbirth, and his amulet was often worn or venerated by women. Dwarf images are found in at least 50 tombs, suggesting they had significant social roles – as jewellery makers, as keepers of the wardrobe, fishermen, entertainers and personal attendants. For example, the dwarf Seneb is known from a magnificent surviving statue of him with his (non-disabled) wife and his two children: he clearly had an important official role in the Pharaoh's household.

Venerated people in myth and legend had impairments. For example, the Greek god Hephaestus (equivalent of Roman god Vulcan) had a deformed foot, as did Oedipus. The poet Homer is traditionally thought to have been blind. Perhaps an even more influential disabled person of the ancient world was the Old Testament prophet Moses, who is said to have had a speech impediment. In Norse myth, the god Odin sacrificed one of his eyes to gain knowledge; his son Höðr was born blind. Like Hephaestus, the legendary Weyland was the smith of the gods – and was lame, because King Niðhad cut his hamstrings to hobble him.

Prominent historical figures with disabilities in the classical period include the Roman Emperor Claudius (10 BC–AD 54), who had a limp and a speech impediment, which probably resulted from cerebral palsy. Despite the scorn of his family, he was a surprisingly successful and reforming Emperor, responsible for the conquest of Britain among other things. Another disabled person who conquered swathes of Britain was the Viking Ivar the Boneless, son of the Danish king Ragnar Lothbrok. Described in the sagas as having 'only the like of gristle where his bones should have been', it's possible he had some form of genetic disease, perhaps Ehlers-Danlos syndrome, which causes very floppy joints, or maybe even osteogenesis imperfecta, brittle bone disease. According to the sagas, he was unable to walk, and either had to be carried around or to use crutches. Despite this, he was also described as cunning and a master of battle strategy. In 865, he and his brothers led the Great Heathen Army to conquer parts of Northumbria and Mercia and East Anglia, including the great cities of York and Nottingham – and to defeat the Anglo-Saxons. Along the way, the saintly King Edmund of East Anglia was martyred. Eventually, King Alfred of Wessex rallied the locals and defeated the Danes. Meanwhile, Ivar had turned his attention to Scotland, before finally dying peacefully in 873.

The reason to recount these stories of legendary or historical figures is to show that disability was not always negative, and high status disabled people were sometimes very successful in the past. Yet these notable individuals should not distract attention from the difficulties most people with impairments would have faced. Negative attitudes to disability are evident both in Greco-Roman culture and the Judaeo-Christian tradition. Although formally the Christian religion forbade infanticide – with children being abandoned at the church door instead of being killed – there was not a greater acceptance of disability as a result. The common medieval idea of the changeling was that devils had substituted their own – presumably impaired or deformed – offspring in place of the human child. The Protestant reformer Martin Luther (1483–1546), who seems to have believed the changeling myth, once advocated that a severely disabled infant be drowned, blaming the devil for the deformity. Paracelsus (1493–1541) regarded people with learning difficulties as the outcome of Adam and Eve's fall from grace. But he also says 'Even if the nature went wrong, yet nothing has been wrong with the soul and with the spirit.'

Turning to the Islamic tradition, Abu 'L'Ala Ahmad ibn 'Abdallah al-Ma'arri (973–1057) was both one of the greatest of Arab poets and a rare example of a Medieval free thinker. He came from an elite family, and he won fame due to his originality and intelligence. He went blind as a child, due to smallpox. Beginning his career as a poet at the age of 11, Al-Ma'aari travelled around the region, to Aleppo, to Antioch, in modern day Turkey, and then to Baghdad, receiving a religious, linguistic and literary education through learning the poetic tradition. His first poetry collection was called *The Tinder Spark*. He went on to create another innovative and radical collection of verse, the *Luzumiyyat*. Translated as 'Unnecessary necessities', the title apparently referred both to his attitude to living, and to the obscure vocabulary and complex structure of his poetry. His third great work was *Risalat-al-Ghufran*, or the 'Epistle of Forgiveness', comparable with Dante's *Divine Comedy*, which it may have influenced. In this poem, the hero visits the Gardens of Paradise, where he meets heathen poets who have found forgiveness.

Al-Ma'arri was controversial in his own time, and is regarded as a heretic today, because he was one of the rare examples of religious scepticism in the Islamic world. For example, he rejected the idea that Islam had a monopoly on truth, suggesting it was simply a matter of geographical accident what faith people adopted. For Al-Ma'arri, reason alone should guide human beings. He was critical of the self-interested and often corrupt edifice of religion. He also opposed all violence and killing, becoming a vegan and avoiding the use of animal skins in clothing and footwear. The life of Al-Ma'arri tells us something of what could be possible for a disabled person in medieval Mesopotamia. He composed his writings entirely in his head, and dictated it to others. He also conducted an extensive correspondence. We know from a Persian poet who visited Al-Ma'arri when he was in his seventies that he was 'the chief man in the town, very rich, revered by the inhabitants and surrounded by more than two hundred students who came from all parts to attend his lectures on literature and poetry'. Al-Ma'arri lived at a time and in a culture where blind people were not necessarily excluded.

TRANSITION FROM AGRARIAN TO CAPITALIST SOCIETIES

Life for ordinary disabled people prior to the modern era was far from easy. In an era before effective education or healthcare or public services, the family was the main source of support. Mortality rates would have been high: a third to a half of all children probably died in infancy, some through neglect, as happens in some developing countries today. Because of high levels of superstition and ignorance, non-disabled people would have been more likely to attribute impairment to witchcraft or perhaps the sins of the parents. Presumably, due to diseases like polio, smallpox, scrofula and other problems, more people would have had visible deformities and disfigurements, so disability would have been part of life. But, conversely, although the incidence of impairment was high, life expectancy was shorter, so overall, the prevalence of impairment may not have been much different from today.

Yet from the disability perspective, the way of life in pre-industrial, pre-capitalist times might have been more inclusive, for those who their survived illness or injury. The household was the unit of production, and everyone contributed, young people and old people, strong people and weak people: everyone could do something to benefit the family. Most people worked on the land. It mattered less if you were illiterate or had communication problems or had learning difficulties, when only the monks and a few of the nobility could read. Most agricultural tasks were simple and were learned by copying others, not by getting educational qualifications.

If you did not work on the land, you might be an artisan, making shoes or clothes or doing other crafts, using hand tools, or making bread or beer. Some disabled people could do some of these jobs, and make a living for themselves, either alone or with other members of their family. For many disabled people, even those with mobility impairments, it would have been possible to make some contribution to this work, not least because most people did not have to travel far to get to work. Many people would never have left their home village. In agrarian societies, whether in medieval Europe or in rural parts of Africa or Asia today, disabled people experience a similar level of poverty or hardship as everyone else. If everyone is working at subsistence levels, and households support all their members, then disabled people may not be as disadvantaged as we might imagine. Really determined individuals can sometimes manage to do very well, as I have found in my research in Africa.

One Englishman with disabilities who we know about from the Early Modern period was Nicholas Owen (1550–1606), possibly a dwarf – certainly extremely short – and with a series of other health problems, such as hernia and a damaged leg. The latter seemed to have resulted when a horse fell on him, and the broken leg was never properly set. The hernia was an injury caused by Owen's rather specialist work. Owen was a Catholic, a lay Jesuit, at a time when his religion was proscribed in England. He was born in Oxford, and apprenticed as a carpenter, like his father Walter, later becoming a servant to Henry Garnett, a Jesuit who employed Owen to do some covert carpentry. Known to other recusants as Little John, Owen travelled around the country by night, and did his work secretly, because he was a builder of priests' holes, secret compartments in the houses of the crypto-Catholic gentry.

Whereas previously, these refuges were no more than holes in the floor, Owen built every one differently, and each more ingeniously than earlier examples. Despite his physical limitations, he laboured with masonry and carpentry and trompe l'oeil effects. Over thirty years, he is known to have built at least 100 priest-holes, expertly hidden from the eyes of Pursuivants (anti-Catholic agents) by false fronts, secret trapdoors, covert stairs or underground passageways. He was arrested several times, for example in 1594, when he was only released after a wealthy Catholic family paid his fine. He was arrested for the last time in Worcestershire in 1606, when anti-Catholic feeling was at a height in the wake of the Gunpowder Plot. Hearing of the capture, one of the Privy Councillors said: 'Is he taken that knows all the secret places? I am very glad of that. We will have a trick for him.'

Nicholas Owen was taken first to the Marshalsea Prison, and then to the Tower of London, where he was tortured on the track, in contravention of the medieval tradition that 'maimed people' were not to be exposed to torture. Nevertheless, Owen named no names: he made a confession of his own activities, but without incriminating anyone else. He died in the Tower on 2 March 1606, disembowelled: the authorities later claimed that he had done the deed himself. A jailor admitted to one of Nicholas Owen's relatives that in fact his hands were so damaged by the end that he could barely feed himself.

In Europe, the transition to industrial capitalism happened by degrees. The land was enclosed by the rich and powerful, and given over to sheep. This created a class of landless labourers, who began to move to the urban areas to find work. Agriculture became more scientific and intensive. There was a shift from hand production of wool and cloth and iron and other necessaries to machine production, leading to economies of scale and cheap, mass-produced goods. Manufactories were created in towns and cities, and were increasingly mechanised. For example, the hand-loom weaver was replaced by the fly shuttle (1738); the spinning jenny was developed in place of the spinning wheel (1764), to ensure a steady supply of yarn for the new looms. In this period, agriculture also became mechanised, with horse-drawn seed-drills (1731) and eventually steam-powered threshing machines (1812). Heavy industries produced the coal and iron and ships which were needed for international trade. People now increasingly worked long hours for a wage, and employers wanted strong, fit young workers, who were able to operate their machines. With formal employment came, for the first time, unemployment.

Disabled people would have been disadvantaged in the quest for paid work. Many would not have been able to work the machines, because many disabled people are not as strong, or as quick, or as cognitively able as non-disabled people. They may not have been able to travel to work, or get into the workplace. Often excluded from higher education, like women, they were excluded from high status jobs in the professions or in commerce. But whereas women either worked on factory production lines, did piece-work (weaving, sewing, etc.) or became teachers, many disabled people would have been unable to take these roles. This left them excluded from the developing capitalist economy. Not only that, but people who would have supported them had themselves been absorbed into wage labour, leaving disabled people without care or help. This was one of the drivers behind institutionalisation.

Very similar processes are operating today, as countries in the developing world become more developed. Economies in sub-Saharan Africa are moving from a high level of informality – for example, self-employment and small businesses and farming – towards increased formality – for example, working for large employers in the formal economy. This means you do not go to an individual tailor or cobbler for your clothes or shoes, you buy mass produced clothing and footwear from a chain store. As a result, the disabled craftspeople lose out. A 'disability and development gap' begins to open up, as non-disabled people prosper as a result of more wage-labour, but disabled people fall behind, for exactly the same reasons as they were disadvantaged by the advent of industrial capitalism in Europe.

FREAK SHOWS

While most people lived by agrarian or craft work, some disabled people have always made a living from their difference, as entertainers or mascots for public exhibition. Jeffrey Hudson (1619–1682) was the son of an Oakham butcher who worked for the Duke of Buckingham, and was brought to the court of King Charles I, where he stepped out of a pie at table, and ended up as a page to Queen Henrietta Maria. He is recorded as having fought duels, and commanded cavalry. Court dwarfs can be seen in paintings by Velasquez and Mantegna, and conjoined twins and other oddities would be brought to the court as entertainment. For example, Matthias Buchinger (1674–1740), 'the little man from Nuremberg', born without hands and feet, who found fame as an artist, musician and conjuror, but tried unsuccessfully to get an audience with King George I. The Russian Tsar Peter the Great was another ruler with a penchant for the unusual. In the Ottoman court, not only dwarfs but also Deaf people were employed in the harem, where they used their own form of sign language.

Right through to the modern era, people with unusual body forms have found employment in fairs and freak shows. In the 1840s, the American showman P. T. Barnum began a tradition with performers such as General Tom Thumb (1838–1883), which continues today in some location such as Coney Island. The nineteenth century was the highpoint of the freak show, with famous individuals such as Joseph Merrick (1862–1890), who found fame as 'The Elephant Man' during the 1880s, and whose story has been memorialised in books and films. Tod Browning's 1932 film *Freaks* features disabled people in a travelling freak show, and explores the romance between a non-disabled woman and one of the stars. It culminates in the circus people taking revenge on the non-disabled woman. The film was considered horrific, banned in the UK, and then lost until re-release in 1962, since when it has been regarded as a cult classic.

Today, while actual freak shows are rare, they have to some extent been replaced by sensational television documentaries and magazine articles about people with unusual bodies or lifestyles, which also meet the same popular desire for titillation. Whether individual disabled people have the right to participate in entertainments which arguably denigrate disabled people as a whole remains a sensitive issue. For example, some people with restricted growth continue to perform in *Snow White and the Seven Dwarfs* and other entertainments such as 'dwarf tossing', where they are figures of fun. Many other restricted growth people find this challenging, even offensive. But in a free society, individuals are able to seek any form of employment, even if this arguably undermines their peers' chances of achieving equal respect or being taken seriously as potential employees.

FROM BEGGARS TO INSTITUTIONS

For those disabled people who had no family to support them, the only option in medieval England was to seek support from a monastery or a charitable almshouse, or to beg. The 1531 Vagabonds Act meant that 'deserving poor' – particularly old or disabled people – were given a licence and an area within which they could beg. Poor rates were subsequently levied on communities to provide funds for supporting impoverished people, including disabled people. The Elizabethan Poor Law of 1601 regularised the system. The deserving 'impotent poor' (old or disabled) were given food ('the parish loaf') and clothing in the system of 'outdoor relief'. From 1700, workhouses began to be constructed in towns and cities, to house both the 'deserving' and 'undeserving' poor. By 1776, there were 1,912 of them. They increasingly became restricted to disabled and older people, with the unemployed forced to work.

By 1834, there were 4800 workhouses in Britain. The 1834 Poor Law Amendment Act not only promoted construction of more workhouses, but also introduced the principle of 'less eligibility', whereby it was made so miserable for people in the workhouse that they would rather work than experience this treatment. The Act also disenfranchised residents of workhouses. Of course, disabled people, who often could not work, were the main victims of this social policy. The abuses of these workhouses were exposed in novels by Dickens and others. At this point, it was less that the destitute had a right to relief, more that the community had an obligation to relieve poverty and promote work. In the late nineteenth century, local authorities were created, and alternatives developed to the workhouse. By 1911, the beginnings of the welfare state were forming. From the 1920s onwards, charities developed residential homes for disabled adults, while local authorities were creating residential accommodation for older people. Yet, for many older people, the stigma of the workhouse and depending on others for your maintenance was still felt.

Turning to mental health history, prior to the nineteenth century, most people with mental illness would have been supported by their families. The Bethlem Royal Hospital in London dates from the early seventeenth century, and the Bethel Hospital in Norwich was opened in 1713. By 1807, there were seventeen small madhouses in London, and only seven significant madhouses outside the capital. This situation changed, when Enlightenment physicians such as Philippe Pinel began to argue that mental illness was a disease, which could be cured, by removing chains, stopping punishment, improving conditions. In England, the Quaker William Tuke created the York Retreat in 1796, where 30 people were able to live without restraints in a comfortable country setting, resting and talking and doing manual work, an approach which was called 'moral treatment'.

After the 1808 Country Asylums Act, magistrates were able to build asylums for 'pauper lunatics'. Twenty years later,

Commissioners in Lunacy were appointed to inspect conditions in asylums. Over the nineteenth century, there was also a huge increase in the creation of lunatic asylums for people with mental health conditions. Those with mild distress would be housed in workhouses, but people with serious mental health problems would be moved on to asylums. From 1853 the Poor Law Commission prohibited the use of chains and manacles. Hundreds of thousands of people became incarcerated, often in over-crowded conditions, with consequent abuses. Despite the optimism of the early reformers, there were no effective treatments for mental illness, until the discovery of anti-psychotic drugs from the 1950s onwards. With better treatments, the movement for reform and de-institutionalisation took off in the 1950s and 1960s.

MANAGING URBAN SPACE

Beggars were unwelcome during the transition to modernity. In nineteenth century America, there was a crop of what should more accurately be called 'unsightly beggar ordinances'. These laws are epitomised by the Chicago ordinance of 1871 which prohibited 'Any person who is diseased, maimed, mutilated or in any way deformed, so as to be an unsightly or disgusting object, or an improper person to be allowed in or on the streets, highways, thoroughfares, or public places in the city...' from exposing themselves, i.e. for the purpose of begging. Starting with San Francisco in 1867, many American cities passed similar ordinances leading up to the first decades of the twentieth century: a society exalting the 'self-made man' was never going to have much time for the impoverished or impaired. While in principle Civil War veterans were regarded as honourable, others were suspected as being inauthentic, or even as having faked their injuries ('sham cripples'). Persecution, fines, and incarceration in the Alms House was the fate of many disabled people in late nineteenth century America. The growth of charitable institu-tions, then as now, was a mixed blessing for the disabled community. What in 1919 one disabled vagrant called 'a hard sanctimoniousness' ruled. For example, many of those who had fought for England and been impaired as a result ended up in residential homes like the Star and Garter Homes, where they were patronised and segregated, and even sometimes treated like children, to their deep frustration.

Even without these extremes, it is important to note that modern cities grew up at a time when disabled people were largely excluded from participation in public life, which meant that their needs did not have to be considered. The great civic buildings of Europe were built on classical lines, with imposing flights of steps. Schools, workplaces and other ordinary buildings were also never designed to be accessible to all who might want to use them. The new forms of mass transport – trains and trams and buses – were constructed with no thought for people with mobility impairments or even children. Centuries later, expensive retro-fitting has been necessary to ensure that access barriers can be minimised with the addition of ramps, lifts and accessible toilets.

A little-known Londoner with disabilities was May Billinghurst (1875–1953), who was born in Lewisham. At five months old, she contracted an illness – probably polio. She was left paraplegic, relying on callipers and crutches to walk, and usually resorting to a hand-pedalled three-wheeler wheelchair. Like many middle-class women of her era, she started doing good works in poor parts of London. But then radicalised by her experiences, in 1907 she joined the militant suffragette Women's Social and Political Union (WSPU) and thereafter became known as 'the cripple suffragette'. Always on her tricycle, decorated with WSPU ribbons and banners, she participated in the suffragette march to the Albert Hall on 13 June 1908, distributing leaflets advertising the forthcoming Hyde Park demonstration. She founded a local branch of the WSPU in Greenwich.

May repeatedly came into contact with the police and the authorities. She would have running battles with the police, charging them in her invalid chair. In November 1910, she was thrown out of her tricycle during the 'Black Friday' demonstration, and the police pushed her down a side street and removed the valves from her tyres. She was one of 159 women arrested that day. A year later, May was arrested again in Parliament Square and sentenced to five days in prison for obstructing the police. In March 1912, she was sentenced to one month's hard labour in

Holloway Prison after smashing windows as part of the WPSU campaign. She had hidden the stones for flinging at windows under the rug over her legs. In December that year, she was sentenced to eight months in prison, after being found guilty of firebombing Deptford pillar boxes. On this last occasion, she went on hunger strike, and was forcibly fed, causing damage to her health and teeth. After many letters of protest, after two weeks her release was ordered by the Home Secretary.

In March 1913, she was able to speak about her experiences at a meeting in West Hampstead. In June 1913, she took part in the funeral procession for Emily Wilding Davison – the suffragette who had flung herself at the King's horse at The Derby and been trampled to death. In her invalid tricycle, as always, May wore white on this occasion. On 21 May 1914, she chained herself and her chair to the railings as Buckingham Palace as part of another WPSU protest.

Once the First World War broke out, WPSU suspended campaigning, and members were released from prison. May supported Christabel Pankhurst's Smethwick election campaign in 1918, the year that the Qualification of Women Act was passed. After this, May ceased to be politically active and little more is known of her, except that she lived in Sunbury on Thames (Surrey) and had an adopted daughter.

EUGENICS AND EUTHANASIA

In the first part of the twentieth century, eugenics was in fashion. The word 'eugenics' was coined in 1883 by Francis Galton, a cousin of Charles Darwin, to mean 'well born'. Galton defined it as 'the science of the improvement of the human germ plasm though better breeding'. Positive eugenics was the encouragement of 'better' sections of society to have more children. Negative eugenic was the opposite: the discouragement or even prohibition of reproduction by 'lesser' sections of society. These policies came in voluntary versions – such as 'Bonnie Baby' competitions – and in compulsory forms, as with the increasing number of countries and regions that mandated involuntary sterilisation of certain sections of the population. This always included so-called 'feeble minded' people – people with learning difficulties – and also often people with epilepsy, schizophrenia and other conditions. Until 1945, eugenics was an intellectual trend on the left and the right. It was adopted as official policy in most developed countries: many American states, the Canadian province of Alberta, Denmark, Finland, Germany, Japan, Norway, Sweden, Switzerland introduced sterilisation laws. In other countries, such as Britain and France, eugenics remained an intellectual movement but never became enshrined in law.

The country that applied a eugenics policy in its most extreme form was Germany. In the 1920s, tracts were being written which celebrated eugenics and even proposed euthanasia. During the 1930s, Nazi propaganda was stigmatising so-called 'useless eaters', 'ballast existence' and 'lives unworthy of life', and promoting 'mercy killing'. In 1933, after the Nazis came to power, the Law for the Prevention of Genetically Impaired Progeny was implemented. This law, which was applauded by American eugenicists, mandated compulsory sterilisation. Between 14 July 1933 and 1 September 1939, approximately 375,000 people with 'feeble-mindedness', schizophrenia, bipolar disorder, epilepsy, Huntington's disease, blindness, deafness, deformity and also severe alcoholism were sterilised. The category 'feeble-minded' was very vague: hereditary health courts asked questions like 'When is Christmas?' and 'Who discovered America?' to distinguish those eligible for the operation. In 1935, the Marriage Health Law prohibited people with mental illness, hereditary disease or contagious disease from marrying.

Finally, at the outbreak of war, the notorious Nazi euthanasia programme began covertly, ordered by Hitler himself. Under the T4 programme, questionnaires were dispatched to all residential institutions. Disabled people were cursorily evaluated by medical experts. A transport office, run by the SS, collected those who had been selected and took them to one of six killing centres. There, in groups of 75 or more, they were stripped and taken for a 'shower', where they were gassed with carbon monoxide. Any gold teeth were removed from the corpses, which were then burned in ovens. By the time this official T4 programme was halted in August 1941, after protests from the Catholic Church and from relatives, at least 70,000 people were killed.

Alongside the official programme, there was children's euthanasia in hospitals all over Germany. Newborns and infants under three with a range of conditions, including spina bifida, dwarfism, Down syndrome, blindness and deafness and other conditions, were registered, evaluated, and then transferred to one of 28 'specialist children's wards', where they were killed with a lethal injection, or an overdose of everyday medications, or even starved to death. At least 5,000 children were killed in this way.

After the end of formal euthanasia, a phase of so-called 'wild euthanasia' took over, where disabled people, elderly people and 'antisocial elements' were killed in a less systematic way. Also, any mentally ill, disabled or long-term care patients were killed in hospitals in the territories to the east which the Nazis were conquering – Russia, Poland, Ukraine. Finally, the T4 organisation was invited to work in the concentration camps, where a further 20,000 people who were unable to work were gassed. This process ended in 1943, by which time the 'Final Solution' of the Jewish inmates of the death camps was well underway. In Auschwitz, the notorious Dr Josef Mengele and others were conducting 'experiments' on disabled Jewish people. During the euthanasia programme, upwards of 275,000 disabled men, women and children were murdered.

Despite revulsion at these Nazi abuses, eugenics ideas and laws continued after 1945. Many university eugenics departments simply changed their name to genetics departments after 1945. While Nazi doctors were tried and executed, and post-war genetics adopted an ethos of informed consent, eugenic thinking has taken longer to be dislodged. For example, Sweden only prohibited the sterilisation of people without consent in 1975. DNA pioneer Francis Crick later suggested people should have to have a licence to have children. In the 1990s, IVF pioneer Dr Robert Edwards said at a conference that in the future, it would be a 'sin' to have a disabled child. Some of the prevailing negative attitudes about disabled people, particularly people with learning difficulties, becoming parents, seem to be a reversion to this eugenic past.

DISABILITY IN POST-WAR BRITAIN

At the end of the war, alongside the 1948 National Health Act and other pillars of the British welfare state, specific legislation addressed the needs of disabled people, particularly those who had been injured in conflict. The National Assistance Act required local authorities to house people who needed support because of age or infirmity. The National Insurance Act of 1946 enshrined a right to incapacity benefit. However, payments were at low levels and hard to access. The 1944 Education Act promoted education for all, but relegated disabled children, in eleven different categories, to special schools. The 1944 Disabled Persons (Employment) Act set a quota of 3 per cent of jobs occupied by disabled people in all large enterprises. The hope was that mainstream employment opportunities would develop for disabled people. However, this Act was largely ignored, and for many years, the main opportunities for employment were in sheltered workshops. Historian Anne Borsay concludes that the rights of disabled people were a low priority within the agenda for rebuilding post-war Britain.

By the 1960s, individuals with disabilities and their families were beginning to agitate for better provision, as the limitations of the post-war settlement became clearer. In 1963, RIBA's *Designing for the Disabled* outlined how buildings could be made more accessible to all. The author was an architect who had survived polio, Selwyn Goldsmith. Labour MP Alf Morris was responsible for the Chronically Sick and Disabled Persons Act, passed in 1970. This legislation compelled local authorities to create a register of disabled people, and to provide services in the community such as home helps and meals on wheels. It also mandated adaptations to housing to improve accessibility. However, these services did not reach everyone who needed them, and the Act was later criticised for empowering professionals, not disabled people.

The exclusion of disabled people, particularly children, found in a response in the growth of the voluntary sector. Charities such as the Royal National Institute of Blind People (founded 1868, became National Institute for the Blind in 1914, changed to current name in 2002) and Action on Hearing Loss (founded in 1911 as Royal National Institute for the Deaf) had tried to support people throughout the twentieth century. But new charities, such as Leonard Cheshire Disability (founded in 1948) and Scope (founded as the National Spastics Society in 1951) grew up in the post-war period. Some of these responses were segregating. For example, there are 270 Cheshire Homes in 49 countries – while undoubtedly helping many people where no other services exist, most disability activists would see residential homes as outdated. Scope started out providing segregated schools, day centres, sheltered workshops and residential institutions. At the time, these were filling a gap, where the state was not providing for disabled children and adults.

The life of Mabel Cooper (1944–2013) illustrates typical experiences of someone with learning difficulties in the twentieth century. She was born in London, where her mother lived on the street. The pair were picked up by the authorities, and sent to institutions, and her mother subsequently disappeared. Mabel spent her childhood in various children's homes. She did not attend school, and consequently did not learn to read and write. Later she was labelled as having learning disability and sent to St Lawrence's Hospital, a long-stay institution in Caterham, Surrey. She later said:

> When I first went in there, even just getting out of the car you could hear the racket. You think you're going to a madhouse. When you first went there you could hear people screaming and shouting outside. It was very noisy, but I think you do get used to them after a little while because it's like everywhere that's big.

After twenty years, Mabel finally left St Lawrence's Hospital in 1977 to live in the community. Later, the hospital was completely closed down, and she was given the honour of pressing the button to blow it up. She was adamant that such institutions should never be allowed in future. Mabel had become an intellectual disability celebrity through her work with Croydon People First, a self-advocacy group. She eventually became chair of London People First. In both roles, she supported other people with learning difficulties to be heard. She collaborated with Dorothy Atkinson and other researchers at the Open University, who helped people with learning difficulties to research and tell their stories as part of the Life History Project. Mabel Cooper's own life story was published in *Forgotten Lives* (1997), and inspired many readers with and without learning difficulties. She went into schools to talk to children and young people about the discrimination and bullying which people with learning difficulties face. She seems to have been a very charismatic person, who used humour to get her points across and changed perceptions about intellectual disability. As recognition for her work, Mabel Cooper was awarded an honorary degree by the Open University in 2010. The inclusion of her obituary in the BBC Radio 4 *Last Word* programme, after she died of cancer in April 2013, is another example of how this ordinary woman with intellectual disability made an extraordinary impact.

During the 1970s, there had been increasing calls for integration, rather than segregation, for example the Snowden Working Party on the Integration of the Disabled, which reported in 1976 (and on which my father, Dr William Shakespeare, served). The chairman, Lord Snowden, was then brother-in-law to the Queen. He had survived polio himself as a child, and retained a limp. Meanwhile, less privileged disabled people resident in institutions such as Cheshire Homes were becoming radicalised and more vocal in their opposition to the dominant paternalistic and exclusionary approach to disability. Even organisations such as the Spastics Society and Cheshire Homes began to change, supporting disabled people to enter the mainstream, rather than keeping them in segregated settings. The name changes which each of these traditional charities have undergone indicate how thinking has modernised. Having disabled people in leadership positions – such as Bill Hargreaves, the first Scope trustee with cerebral palsy – helped create this more empowering approach.

Another landmark was the 1978 Warnock Report, the findings of a commission looking at special education for children with physical or learning difficulties. Between 1945 and 1972, the number of children attending special schools had risen from 38,499 to 106,367. The Warnock Committee recommended abolishing different categories, and thinking of special educational needs on a continuum. The underlying philosophy was one of integration. It influenced the 1981 Education Act, which stated that education of disabled children should be in mainstream schools where possible, with a child supported by a learning support teacher.

CONCLUSION

In this chapter, I have only been able to illuminate some key moments in the history of disability. I am conscious that I have been unable to tell a coherent story. This is partly due to lack of space, although another major obstacle to telling the story of disabled people through the ages is lack of evidence. Historians are only now turning their attention not just to the experience of disabled people, but also the social and economic disabling factors which influenced their lives. In previous centuries, 'disability' was not understood as a separate and distinct category, and nor would disabled people necessarily have thought of themselves as different. As society changed – with factors such as urbanisation and industrialisation – so the lives of people with impairments changed. Modernity, with the advent of scientific medicine, brought huge improvements, but at the cost of segregation.

Meanwhile, notable historical individuals from Horatio Nelson to John Milton to Harriet Martineau undoubtedly had significant impairments, and nevertheless contributed hugely not only to their age but to all time. To me, these great lives show us what disabled people can achieve, given the chance, and given the personal motivation. But equally important are the hidden lives of those who were incarcerated in institutions, or who struggled to survive in the community, and of whom we can only learn scraps and rumours.

FURTHER READING

Robert Bogdan. 2007. *Freak Show: presenting human oddities for amusement and profit.* Chicago, IL: University of Chicago Press.

Anne Borsay. 2005. *Disability and Social Policy in Britain since 1750.* Basingstoke: Palgrave Macmillan.

Susan Burch and Michael Rembis, editors. 2014. *Disability Histories.* Urbana, IL: University of Illinois Press.

Lennard Davis. 1995. *Enforcing Normalcy: disability, deafness and the body.* London: Verso.

Anne Kerr and Tom Shakespeare. 2002. *Genetic Politics: from eugenics to genome.* Cheltenham: New Clarion Press.

Paul Longmore and Lauri Umansky, editors. 2001. *The New Disability History: American perspectives.* New York: New York University Press.

Roddy Slorach. 2016. *A Very Capitalist Condition: a history and politics of disability*. London: Bookmarks.

Rosemarie Garland Thomson, editor. 1996. *Freakery: cultural spectacles of the extraordinary body*. New York: New York University Press.

TIMELINE

1760	Abbé de l'Épée founds a school in Paris to teach sign language to deaf people
1750	Joseph Heath introduces the bath chair, an early wheelchair
1796	William Tuke opens the York Retreat, a more humane asylum for people experiencing mental illness
1817	American School for the Deaf is founded in Hartford, Connecticut
1824	Louis Braille develops his system of tactile writing for blind people
1864	Edward Gallaudet opens college for Deaf people in Washington, DC
1883	Francis Galton coins the word 'eugenics'
1887	Helen Keller, deaf-blind, meets her new tutor, Annie Sullivan
1898	Miller Reese Hutchison invents an electrical hearing aid
1907	Indiana becomes first US state to pass a eugenic sterilisation law
1925	Samuel Orton begins studying dyslexia
1927	Philip Drinker and Louis Shaw develop the iron lung for victims of polio
1932	Everest and Jennings introduce tubular frame folding wheelchair
1932	Franklin Delano Roosevelt elected president for the first of four terms
1943	Leo Kanner of Johns Hopkins Hospital uses the term 'autism' to describe similar behaviour characteristics of 11 young people
1948	Lithium begins to be used as a treatment for bipolar disorder

1950	Chloropromazine, the first pharmaceutical treatment for schizophrenia discovered
1952	Worst recorded polio epidemic (killed 3,145 people)
1955	Salk polio vaccine developed
1957	Thalidomide being marketed as a treatment for morning sickness
1961	Growing awareness of congenital impairments as a result of thalidomide
1962	Ed Roberts, survivor of polio, enrols at University of California, Berkeley
Late 1960s	Amniocentesis introduced for prenatal diagnosis of Down syndrome
1972	Alf Morris MP appointed as Britain's first Minister for Disabled People
1973	US Rehabilitation Act, of which Section 504 prohibited discrimination against people with disabilities in Federal programmes
1976	First cochlear implant operation performed on a deaf man at Sainte-Antoine Hospital in Paris
1979	Quickie lightweight wheelchair created for disabled sportswoman Marilyn Hamilton by her friends Jim Okamoto and Don Helman
1981	International year of disabled people
1984	Serum screening for Down syndrome introduced
1988	'Deaf President Now' campaign at Gallaudet University, USA
1990	Americans with Disabilities Act outlaws discrimination in USA
1995	UK Disability Discrimination Act
2003	Human Genome published
2006	UN adopts Convention on the Rights of Persons with Disabilities

A LIFE WORTH LIVING

This chapter is about how individuals live with impairment and disability. Here again, it is all about diversity. Individual disabled people have different experiences and feel differently about their lives. But there are some generalisations that seem largely true. A key distinction is between those who are born with an impairment and those who acquire one. People disabled from birth are likely to feel that disability is part of their identity. They cannot imagine life without it. They do not have a struggle to 'come to terms'. The idea of being cured of their impairment may be alien and unwelcome. However, they may have to struggle to access education, employment and relationships. They may have poor self-esteem, if they are not brought up to feel positive about themselves.

Conversely, those who acquire disability later in life are in some ways advantaged. They may have already received a good education, they may have a family and a career, and they may have good self-esteem. But acquiring an illness or impairment through trauma or disease usually comes as a major shock. They always thought of disabled people as 'other' and inferior, perhaps. Now they are becoming someone they always felt sorry for. They can no longer do all the things they took for granted. They are often very keen to find a treatment or cure for their condition.

So, depending on the age that disability affects the individual, it is experienced very differently. In this chapter, having said a bit more about quality of life, I will take a life course approach, discussing disability in children, in working-age people, and in older people. In between these sections, I will try and look at some important cross cutting issues –becoming disabled, independent living, and finally violence and abuse. Throughout the chapter, it should be remembered that different impairments have very different consequences for people's lives and prospects: cognitive impairment is not the same as physical impairment, for example.

QUALITY OF LIFE

Impairment seems, on the face of it, a very unpleasant phenomenon, which most people would prefer to avoid. You might hear people saying things like 'I'd rather be better be dead than disabled'. Disability, in everyday thought, is associated with failure, with dependency and with not being able to do things. We feel sorry for disabled people, because we imagine it must be so miserable to be disabled.

But in fact we are usually wrong. Both empirical evidence and anecdotal testimony reveals that for many people with disabilities, life is surprisingly good. The so-called 'disability paradox' refers to the data that reveal how people with disabilities consistently report a quality of life as good as, or sometimes even better than, that of non-disabled people.

Impairment can make little difference to quality of life. The research shows, for example, that overall levels of life satisfaction for people with spinal cord injury are not affected by their physical ability or limitations. Even the clinical fact of whether their spinal lesion is high or low, complete or incomplete – all aspects that affect functioning – doesn't make much difference. Human flourishing is possible even if you lack a major sense, or you can't walk, or you're totally physically dependent on others. So what is going on?

If you think about it for a moment, you realise that people born with an impairment have nothing with which they can compare their current existence. Someone lacking hearing or sight has never experienced music or birdsong, visual art or a sublime landscape. Someone with intellectual disability may not consider themselves different at all. Someone like me, born with restricted growth has always been that way. Even if life is sometimes hard, we are used to being the way we are.

People who become disabled tend to go through a similar trajectory. Immediately after onset of injury or disease, they may feel profoundly depressed, and may even contemplate suicide. Yet after a period of time, they adapt to their situation, re-evaluate their negative attitude to the disability, and start making the most of it. Often they are driven to greater achievements than before. Usually, their quality of life returns to approximately what it was before the trauma struck. This phenomenon, which also explains why lottery winners revert to their previous state of happiness after the thrill of riches has worn off, is known as *hedonic adaptation*.

Bioethicists sometimes describe these self-reports in terms of the 'happy slave' idea, in other words, people think they are happy because they do not know any better. Perhaps these cheerful people with disabilities are deluding themselves. Or perhaps they are deluding others. Maybe in private they admit to misery, while in public they put on a brave face. Either way, commentators suggest, these people must be in denial. But these explanations do not seem entirely reasonable. They are patronising, not to say insulting. And in fact, psychological research has supported disabled people's self- reports of good quality of life. So we need to find better ways of understanding the paradox.

First, we can offer less demeaning explanations of the psychological processes that go on in the mind of a person with disability. *Adaptation* means finding another way to do something: for example, the paralysed person might wheel rather than walk places. *Coping* is when people redefine their expectations about functioning over time. They decide that a stroll of half a mile is fine, whereas previously they would only have been content with a ten miles ramble. *Accommodation* is when someone learns to value other things: they decide that rather than going for walks in the country with friends, it's far more important to be able to go to great restaurants with them. In these ways, over time, people come to terms with their limitation. This teaches us an important lesson: it appears that human beings are capable of adapting to almost any situation, finding satisfaction in the smaller things they can achieve, and deriving happiness from their relationships with family and friends, even in the absence of other triumphs.

Second, our appraisal of life with impairment may have less to do with actuality than with fear and ignorance and prejudice, all of which make the experience appear worse than it actually is. We have a distorted view of disability, made more graphic by the ways cultural representations of disability play on our anxiety about incapacity, and dependency. The imagination is a dangerous tool when it comes to disability: we tend to exaggerate, project, and mistake what life is really like for people with disabilities. We wrongly assume that difficulties for people result in misery for people.

Even to the extent that health conditions and impairments do entail suffering and limitation, other factors in life can more than compensate for them: for example, an individual with access to resources, such as Philippe, the protagonist of the 2011 French box office sensation *Les Intouchables* can have an extremely good quality of life notwithstanding his tetraplegia – the film was based on the true story of Philippe Pozzo di Borgo and his French–Algerian caregiver Abdel Sellou. The theoretical physicist Stephen Hawking has numerous personal assistants and all the technology he needs to do his science – he too is the subject of a major Hollywood film, *The Theory of Everything*. Even someone who is not lucky enough to be a wealthy Parisian aristocrat or an award-winning scientist can enjoy the benefits of friendship or culture, notwithstanding the restrictions that impairment places on her. By contrast, it is plain to see that someone can have a fully functioning body or mind and yet lack the social networks or the personality necessary for living a happy and fulfilled existence.

This highlights the importance of the environment in determining the happiness of disabled people. Evidence shows that impairment is not the key issue. As in most areas of life, it's structural factors that make the real difference for disabled people. Do access barriers stop you going to school with your friends? Do you have a job? Does society meet the extra costs of having an impairment via a welfare system which is fair and non-stigmatising? Do you face hostility and hate crime? In Chapter 4, I will discuss these social barriers in greater depth.

In asserting that environmental barriers can be more of a problem than the impairment itself, I am not suggesting that it is completely irrational to fear disability. For a start, disability is very diverse in ways that mean we have to qualify the claim that 'disability is no tragedy'. Some illnesses and impairments undoubtedly involve greater degrees of misery and suffering than the average human should have to endure. For example, unipolar and bipolar depression, which Lewis Wolpert memorably labelled 'malignant sadness'. There are some nasty and painful degenerative diseases. People who experience these conditions will certainly have periods of happiness and fulfilment. They can enjoy many aspects of life. But overall, it is much harder to be sanguine about these forms of life than it is about impairments such as deafness. Discussions of the 'disability paradox' are often qualified with the observation that impairments that involve considerable pain, whether physical or mental, are less compatible with a good quality of life.

It's also true that in general, disabled people usually have fewer choices than non-disabled people. Most societies still have sub-optimal accessibility. Even in a barrier-free world, the disabled person is more likely to rely on mechanical devices – elevators, wheelchairs, communication devices – that periodically malfunction, rendering the individual excluded or dependent. Most disabled people become inured to the frustrations of inaccessibility or breakdown, but it certainly makes life less predictable and less free than non-disabled people take for granted.

While disability is not simply an irrelevant difference like the colour of your skin, neither is it a tragedy. We might instead call it a *predicament*: something we have to come to terms with. We should also remember that mere existence entails problems. Hamlet, listing reasons why death is to be preferred, highlights 'the thousand natural shocks that flesh is heir to'. To be born is to be vulnerable, to fall prey to disease and pain and suffering, and ultimately to die. Even the good life contains difficulties. It would be fantastical to imagine a person whose life was free of any hardship. Sometimes, the part of life that is difficult brings other benefits, such as a sense of perspective or true value that people who lead easier lives can miss out on. Disability is not defined by frailty and vulnerability, because life itself is about frailty and vulnerability. If we always remembered this truth about life, perhaps we would turn out to be more accepting of disability and a little less prejudiced against disabled people.

DISABILITY IN CHILDHOOD

Health conditions associated with disability are rarer in childhood than at later stages of life. Genetic conditions such as muscular dystrophy, cystic fibrosis or my own condition, achondroplasia (dwarfism) are very uncommon. For example, achondroplasia occurs about once in every 20,000 births. Cerebral palsy, usually mainly resulting from lack of oxygen during labour, has an incidence of one in 400 births. In total, approximately 1–2 per cent of all births are affected by some form of congenital impairment. Nearly half of all premature babies have some form of impairment, although this number is declining. Other impairments – such as autistic spectrum conditions – become evident in the second or third year of life, as children fail to make expected developmental milestones. Finally, accidents are a major cause of impairment in young people. In total, approximately 5 per cent of children are disabled.

Data also show that more boys than girls have disabilities. Disabled children are more likely to be in single parent families, and more likely to have a parent who is also disabled. There is a strong correlation between childhood disability and poverty. This is partly because families in poverty are more likely to have a disabled child, but also because when there is a disabled child to look after, it is very common for one parent to give up work to care for that child, resulting in financial hardship for the family.

When a newborn or infant is diagnosed with a health condition such as Down syndrome or muscular dystrophy or autism, the way that the news is communicated is very important. Doctors may feel uncomfortable 'breaking bad news'. They may lack training or competence in talking to patients. Some hospitals have a tacit policy of doctors being accompanied by nurses when communicating diagnoses, because the nurses are better at dealing with people. Diagnosis can be a process rather than an event – extensive investigations may take weeks or even months. But although stressful, diagnosis can be a relief to parents, who are aware something is different about their child, but worried about what it might be.

Disability impacts differently at different stages of development. As babies, there may be little difference: all babies are dependent and demanding. But when children begin to be able to walk, often disabled children still need to be carried – perhaps even when they are much older. When children start communicating, some disabled children are less able to interact. When children start school, it is often the first time they realise they are different. Other children stare at them, and sometimes they are bullied. Getting their son or daughter into a school where they will be safe, and where they will receive any support that is required, is the major goal for parents of a disabled child. Then again, when teenage children start becoming independent, disabled children may again fail to grow away from their parents and carers. While other young people are thinking about jobs, college and careers, parents of disabled people may be worrying about the transition from paediatric to adult services, and fearing for their child's future.

Ways of thinking about disabled children are often very negative. Phrases like burden, loss and grief are common in the literature. Most of the research is not done with children themselves, it is done with their parents, carers or professionals. The common reaction to hearing about a child with disabilities is pity or sympathy. For parents too, the first reaction is often grief and other complex emotions – guilt, shame, anger, sadness. It can take a year or more to come to terms with the birth of a disabled child. The way a diagnosis is communicated can be essential to how families adapt, as we will discuss in Chapter 5. Coping can be difficult, because of factors such as lost sleep, exhaustion and back pain, emotional strain.

Parents have to develop expertise in negotiating with the maze of services and managing professionals in fields like health, rehabilitation, assistive technology, education, social services. Evidence shows that parents have to fight for appropriate services. Often, the interface between health and social services is rigid and inflexible. Entitlements may be unclear, and there can be a post-code lottery between different regions of the country. When assessments are needed – for services or welfare benefits – this means focusing on what is wrong with the child, which can feel very negative. Parents often end up paying for needed equipment or spend more money on laundry or transport.

But there is a danger of pathologising too much, and of emphasising difference. When you talk with disabled children – as my research team did in the 1990s – you find that they reject the label of disabled. They just want to be seen and treated like other children. They think of themselves as children first, and disabled second: 'You should go beyond disability and look at the person inside' said one; 'I just try to ignore it and join in' said another. It is vital to change attitudes to disabled children, replacing pity and sorrow with equal treatment. Disabled children have the same needs and issues as non-disabled children. Moreover, big studies of the quality of life of children with cerebral palsy, for example, find that they have similar quality of life to non-disabled children on almost all domains – except schooling, where they do better, and physical well-being, where they do worse. These findings are echoed in studies with children with mobility impairment or spina bifida. However, there is an association between pain and lower quality of life, which is probably why there is an association between severity of juvenile arthritis and poorer quality of life.

Social barriers are big issues in the lives of disabled children, not just individual or health factors. Medical care has a role, but disabled children's lives should not always be dominated by medicine. Sometimes, it is important to know when not to pursue the medical path. For example, a study of families applying for financial assistance from the Family Fund Trust found that both impairment and environmental factors affected participation to similar extents. Support, physical activity and transport were the major factors that affected participation. For example, children with disabilities may be unable to go on school trips, if transport or accommodation is inaccessible; they are very likely to be unable to visit other school friends in their own homes. Negative attitudes also represent barriers – such as the other parents who may not invite the disabled child to the party, or the strangers who pass judgement on the parents when the child with learning difficulties 'misbehaves' in public.

Another important phase is transition from child to adult. Other children may expect to go off to university at age 18 or 19. This may not be an option for the young person who has complex health needs, particularly learning difficulties. Similarly, they may be less likely to leave home and find a job. At this age, disabled young people transition from paediatric services – which may be very personalised and specific to the health issues – to adult services, in which they may feel abandoned and unsupported. They will have to claim welfare benefits in their own rights, rather than these being claimed by the parents. Various service interventions have sought to bridge this gap, such as transition assessments, transition plans, transition coordinators. Transition may be particularly uncertain for young people who have limited life expectancies. In past decades, young men with Duchenne Muscular Dystrophy, for example, would have not survived their teenage years. Now, thanks to better medical treatment, they are living till 25 or beyond, which makes questions of sexuality and employment more important.

Families with disabled children are both similar and different to other families. For example, there may be impacts on siblings. They may get less attention. They may have a role in caring for the disabled child, or in protecting them from bullying at school. Their parents may be more tired and stressed than other parents. They may lack opportunities to do 'normal' family things. They may even feel guilt at being non-disabled. But they also can benefit from growth of insight and compassion. They develop skills, and take pride in their success. Many people who later have careers working with disabled people turn out to have had a disabled sibling or parent or child. Similarly the majority of parents do achieve equilibrium and cope. Even though their life may be somewhat restricted, they feel satisfied. Above all, they feel love and pride in their disabled children: as one study was titled, 'we're tired but not sad'. The positive aspect of acceptance and achieving perspective comes through in the parent who said to a researcher 'I would be happy to have another autistic child. They are lovely kids. They're really taught me something. They've taught me to look at people in different ways'.

Families of disabled children need to connect with other parents and families who share similar experiences. Peer support is particularly important to non-disabled parents, who are encountering illness or impairment for the first time. Voluntary organisations often support these get-togethers, as well as putting parents in touch with relevant medical experts on their child's rare condition. Parents often develop huge knowledge and expertise, whereas their local doctors may be generalists who do not know much about the health issues. This means a partnership model often develops between parents and professionals. Professionals need to support the family's ability to cope, and the mother and father staying together. Often, men leave their wives when a disabled child is born, particularly in developing countries. If a family does not cope with their disabled child, it is more likely to be hospitalised or taken into care. Therefore it is vital to support the family to function effectively, to share knowledge, and to develop trust.

BECOMING DISABLED

How one is regarded by others and how one feels about oneself are often, usually perhaps, different things. Thus, an individual who would by many be classified as disabled may not feel disabled himself, or may not identify as such. So there is a difference between objective and subjective status. Being and becoming disabled is complex, as my own story illustrates.

People have asked me 'when did you first realise you were disabled?' Growing up in a family with a disabled father, I took the difference we shared for granted. My mother and brother were not disabled, but this seemed natural too. When I first went to school, I felt different. Each time I went to a new school, I was made to feel aware of my difference, because I was an oddity, at least until people got used to me. Through life, one continues to feel ordinary, oneself, not different. You are reminded of your difference when you come through a door and the stranger jumps out of their skin because they were not expecting someone disabled. You are reminded of your difference when a group of children start laughing at you. I truly realised I was disabled when I started having back problems in my twenties.

When I became paralysed at the age of 42, I discovered I was disabled all over again, and now differently, because for the first time I was dependent.

So 'becoming disabled' is not one thing, a sudden change of status. It is a continual process of becoming, of changing, of realising, of identifying and not-identifying. Earlier, I mentioned the research we conducted with disabled children aged 11–16, who did not consider themselves disabled. Ten years later, when we did another project with people with restricted growth, they did not automatically consider themselves disabled either. To begin with, they said to us that they were different, not disabled. Only when their health problems began to impinge, in their thirties and forties, did they consider themselves disabled. I could identify with that!

A key moment for many disabled people is when they meet other disabled people. This may be through a residential school, or a self-help group for people with the same impairment, or a disability rights group or a sporting club. Sometimes it is very disturbing to meet other people with the same condition as you. I have experienced people with restricted growth crossing the road so as not to meet me. Some people would never go to a gathering of people with the same condition as themselves. But for others, it can be a liberating experience to be with other people who share your experience, for the first time.

Most people do not have other family members who share the same impairment, so this affiliation with strangers who share the same health condition is very important. People can gain mutual support and understanding. They can share strategies and solutions for coping with the difficulties that impairment – and disabling environments – can generate. I remember when I developed spinal cord injury and became a wheelchair user. One of my close friends had gone through spinal cord injury rehabilitation, and was able to offer support. Another explained to me how to take the wheels off and then lift your wheelchair into your car on your own. Often, when I meet another wheelchair user, we compare wheelchairs, or talk about where to park, or which shops or pubs are accessible in town. We have an automatic connection which we otherwise would not have. The writer Andrew Sullivan, in his book *Far From the Tree*, about families where children are different from parents, calls this horizontal identity.

WORKING-AGE DISABILITY

Approximately one in ten working-age people are disabled. Most people's goals in life could be summarised as a job, a partner and a family. Disabled people are no different. Employment will be discussed in the next chapter, which leaves relationships and family to talk about here.

Adulthood, particularly young adulthood, is the time that people explore their sexuality, form relationships, and have children. In principle, there is no reason that disabled people cannot enjoy those parts of life on the same basis as others, and many people do. Yet society still retains some prejudices and much ignorance around disabled sexuality. For example, parents may shield young adults with learning difficulties from learning about sexuality. Sex education may not be available to disabled people in special schools. Those who live in residential settings may not have the privacy or the permission to engage in sexual activity. Depending on the country, young people with learning difficulties may be subjected to involuntary contraception or even sterilisation, in order to avoid the risk of conceiving a child. At the same time, evidence shows that disabled people, particularly those with learning difficulties, are disproportionately vulnerable to sexual abuse and violence.

Even without these barriers and abuses, it may still be a challenge for some disabled people to meet partners and enjoy a sexual life. People may feel that they are unattractive and undesirable. They may lack confidence to meet people, or lack the money to buy nice clothes and participate in leisure activities. Disabled people are more likely to be excluded from higher education and employment, which are the settings in which many people meet their partners. The evidence from our study of people with restricted growth was that our respondents were more likely to be single, and more likely to partner at a later age than non-disabled people. Those with complex and profound impairments may struggle to meet partners at all. People with serious mental health conditions often have difficulties with personal relationships: they are more likely to lack friends and to find it hard to sustain partnerships. Moreover, psychotropic drugs which combat depression or schizophrenia often have negative effects on libido or cause weight gain, damaging self-confidence.

Yet despite these intrinsic and extrinsic obstacles, the evidence from Britain and from across the world shows that most disabled people do form partnerships, and many have children. In recent years, the internet has enabled more people to meet others. People with restricted growth often partner with someone else with the same condition. Non-disabled people's marriages may break up when one partner has a traumatic injury, but later new relationships are formed, which may be more sustainable. Older people who become disabled through old age generally stick together and support each other. Today, there is also more support available for disabled parents.

So far, discussion has centred on disabled people as they grow up. But adulthood is a time when many more people become disabled. For working-age adults, typical health conditions associated with disability include the consequences of traumatic injuries, such as spinal cord injury and acquired brain injury. Acquiring impairments can be a major challenge to identity. Having grown up as non-disabled, a young man who breaks his back in a motorbike crash or falls off scaffolding, or a middle-aged woman who develops symptoms of multiple sclerosis, or a man or woman who has a stroke, all have to go through a process of adjustment to a different body and to a different way of being in the world and relating to others. Drawing on research with people with rheumatoid arthritis, the medical sociologist Mike Bury has called this process 'biographical disruption'. Onset may be sudden, or may be insidious, but either way a process of readjustment is required, particularly if any ongoing dependency is involved. Uncertainties about the future and about recovery are particularly hard to cope with. People often ask 'Why me?' or 'Why now?'. Research shows that subjective quality of life can plummet after acquiring impairment; but generally it returns to what it was before, once someone has come to terms, set new goals and resumed ordinary life.

For those who become disabled through injury, but also for others with impairments, rehabilitation can be a major issue. This covers physiotherapy, occupational therapy, speech and language therapy, and assistive devices, together with rehabilitation medicine and other medical and surgical specialisms which try to restore functioning. Time spent in rehabilitation hospitals or spinal injury units can be stressful, lonely and difficult. As well as re-learning physical functions – using a wheelchair, or an orthotic or prosthetic – and possibly speech, the individual probably has to learn how to ask for help, how to manage impaired bladder and bowels, and how to manage sexual functioning. Typically, many people enter rehabilitation with unrealistic goals: for example, the spinal cord injured person may vow to beat paraplegia and walk again. As the weeks go on, an individual comes to terms with what has happened, modifies goals, and eventually accepts his or her bodily limitations. As well as health professionals, the role of self-help groups and disabled role models is particularly important in enabling the individual to realise that life goes on, and that they can resume most of the previous activities which they valued.

Depression and other mental health issues are one of the highest contributors to years lived with disability, and may impact particularly in mid-life. At this stage of life, symptoms of rarer conditions such as multiple sclerosis also may begin to impact functioning. Towards the end of working life, conditions such as osteoarthritis may be increasingly disabling, particularly for people working in manual occupations. Importantly, those born with conditions such as cerebral palsy and restricted growth may find that they age earlier than others, as joint or back pains increasingly limit their functioning. People ageing with existing impairment may well have to retire earlier, which can lead to a loss of social networks as well as a decline in income. While secondary conditions and premature ageing can be difficult, it is also the case that by the time people have reached their fifties or sixties, most non-disabled people have experience of bodily limi-tations, and so disabled people may feel less different and more normal.

Intermittent and fluctuating health conditions – for example, depression and other mental illnesses, or multiple sclerosis or other chronic conditions which can flare up – generate a particular set of difficulties. As these conditions are often invisible, work mates and family members may not be as under-standing and forgiving of difficulties in functioning. Employers may be unwilling to be flexible, when it comes to workers being hospitalised very suddenly or taking time off unpredictably. Although workers have legal rights, as we will see in the next chapter, they may still suffer discrimination.

INDEPENDENT LIVING

With community care reforms in the 1980s, many more disabled people left residential institutions to live in the community. Disabled people's organisations which had been founded to campaign for inclusion now increasingly took on roles as providers of advice and support services. Following the principle of 'nothing about us without us', disabled people's organisations and self-advocacy groups have gained a greater voice in in planning and provision of services, as well as in health and social research.

Personal assistance is a model of support which was pioneered by the disability rights community in the 1970s. Rather than depending on institutional support, or family support, or waiting at home for local authority carers to come on their rounds, personal assistance means that the individual receives direct payments to employ their own support workers. This is liberating. The link between physical dependency and social dependency is broken. The disabled person no longer has to feel grateful, or to be at the whim of their care provider. Because they are now the employer, they are in control. They can receive assistance how they want, when they want, from whom they want.

Within the social care system, the process of direct payments for personal assistance means that the person's needs are assessed by local authority social workers, and then they are given the money directly to pay for their own support workers, or personal assistants. Initially, this direct payment could only legally be managed via the Independent Living Fund charity, because public money could not be disbursed directly to individuals. But from 1996, when the law changed, direct payments to individuals became legal and have since been the preferred method of support for tens of thousands of disabled people in Britain. The model can also be found in all the Nordic countries, in the Netherlands, in Switzerland and in other developed nations.

People feel they are in control, if they can dictate how they are supported. Personal assistants can help disabled people fulfil their caring role as parents – they can also help them become more productive at work. Marriage and other relationships may go better, when a paid assistant is taking on the care tasks, or helping with the chores. Many disabled people describe their personal assistants as their 'arms and legs' – able to do the task they cannot do, but without the disabled person having to feel grateful all the time. For some other disabled people, who may be isolated, having a personal assistant also brings friendship – albeit paid friendship – and companionship in everyday life.

However, many people, particularly older people, still receive homecare, sometimes from local authority staff but more often from private agencies. For example, if you live in rural areas, it can be difficult to recruit personal assistants, and so an agency is a more reliable fall-back. In other cases, disabled people do not want the perceived hassle of becoming an employer and processing pay-roll, even though there are intermediary organisations – particularly disabled people's organisations – who can provide those services. Since the global financial crisis, policies of austerity, for example in Britain, have led to cut-backs to services. Local authorities budgets have been cut by around 30 per cent. As a consequence, disabled people may be awarded fewer hours of support. Rather than being helped to participate in society, they may only be entitled to enough assistance to get up in the morning, have a sponge bath, a sandwich lunch, and a hot supper. Even in the Nordic countries, stricter entitlements has led to fewer people getting support through personal assistance.

The success of personal assistance led to the policy of personalisation being extended further with personal budgets: in this approach, an assessment is made of the needs of an individual, who receives an allocation to pay for them to choose what they want, rather than in the past where they would receive a place at a day-centre or other services. This is intended to increase the control people have over their lives. For people with mild to moderate learning disabilities, it appears that the outcomes have been generally positive. However, where the budget is constrained, and where there is a limited menu of options, it is debatable as to whether the outcomes are improved. Critics claim that the policy motivation may be as much about reducing the costs of social care as enhancing the lives of disabled people.

DISABILITY IN OLDER AGE

As people pass retirement age, health conditions associated with impairment multiply. Half of all disabled people are aged over 60. Whereas medicine has succeeded in reducing mortality – meaning that people live longer – there has been no corresponding success in reducing morbidity – which means that people are likely to be living with disability. Conditions such as stroke, arthritis and rheumatism, and eventually dementia are big causes of functional limitation in older people. People with learning difficulties or other long-term conditions are living longer. However, this important group of people are not well represented in the disability movement or in disability research.

Because impairment is associated with ageing, it may be seen as natural and inevitable. Unlike with younger disabled people, there may not be a positive identity as a disabled person. People may not know about services, or seek help when it is required. Some social services, such as personal assistance, are not available to older disabled people because they are not expected to be part of society. In wider society, attitudes to ageing are very negative, and this ageism can restrict opportunities to develop a positive sense of self.

Yet in coming years, surely this negativity around ageing will have to diminish. Older people will make up a larger and larger proportion of the population. Not least in order to reduce dependency and save health and social care costs, but more positively in order to promote human rights and participation, older disabled people will have to be supported to be active and independent.

People who have been independently living with disability all their lives will not tolerate being excluded, and may be able to share strategies and attitudes with other people who are becoming disabled in later life. A human rights approach to ageing – including a human rights approach to dementia – means respecting the individuality of older people, ensuring that they do not face unnecessary barriers, and removing prejudice. The World Health Organization promotes a network of 'age-friendly cities', using a similar 'barrier-removal' approach that is familiar from the access campaigns of the disability movement.

Informal care is a major issue in the lives of older people. Partners may be looking after their spouses, or younger adults may be looking after their ageing parents. Disabled people themselves make up a large proportion of informal carers – usually one older person with disability looking after another, more severely affected older partner. This is the age group where men suddenly become carers in their own right. Because most people want to live in their own homes, the availability of unpaid care from family members, supported by voluntary and statutory services, is a critical issue. Yet informal carers can often feel isolated and unsupported. They do not want their aged relative taken off their hands, because that would make them feel guilty. But they do need support services. Provision of day services, homecare, information and support can make the whole care system work better, offering family members a break and time for themselves.

Despite informal care, many frail older people do end up in care homes at the end of their lives. Here the challenge is to provide supportive care which does not demean older persons. It seems hard for carers to resist infantilising dependent older people, for example, calling them by diminutives and patronising them. Sadly, there have also been cases of elder abuse, where either formal or informal carers hit people or neglect them, if they become demanding or difficult, or where the strain of providing care becomes too much. Therefore it seems vital to remember that older people are individuals with rights, who have had life times of productive work or homemaking, and who retain knowledge and wisdom. Making space for people to speak for themselves, and be listened to, is one way to capture this.

VIOLENCE AND ABUSE

As Katharine Quarmby's 2011 book *Scapegoat* demonstrated, in recent years there has been a series of truly appalling crimes in Britain, where individuals with disabilities or their families have been harassed over a long period of time. To take some recent examples: in 2007 Fiona Pilkington killed both her daughter and herself, after years of being harassed to the point of desperation. In 2010, David Askew, a 64-year-old man with learning difficulties from Greater Manchester, collapsed and died after years of bullying from local youths, who would prey on him for money and cigarettes. In 2012, an enquiry was set up to investigate the widespread and ongoing abuses of people with learning difficulties at Winterbourne View, after undercover reporting at the private 'care home' by the BBC *Panorama* programme. Six members of staff went to prison as a result of criminal proceedings.

There are many examples of people with learning difficulties who have been befriended and preyed on for their welfare benefits or for somewhere to stay – so called 'mate crime' – before in some cases being tortured and murdered. Furthermore, most people with learning difficulties can describe acts of physical violence committed against them by non-disabled people – such as the individual who told me about being tied to a tree and urinated on by young people. Back in 2000, the Mencap *Living in Fear* report showed that bullying was ubiquitous in the lives of people with learning difficulties: 90 per cent said they had been bullied in previous 12 months, and 23 per cent had been assaulted.

People with other impairments can commonly list dozens of instances when they have been called names, stared at or otherwise mocked or bullied by non-disabled people, and some have experienced physical violence. 62 per cent of British young people responding to a 2012 Muscular Dystrophy Campaign survey had been taunted or verbally abused because they were disabled. The research that my team conducted with people with restricted growth in the north of England found that:

- **96 per cent** of respondents had experienced staring or point-ing;
- **77 per cent** had been on the receiving-end of verbal abuse;
- **75 per cent** felt they often attract unwanted attention;
- **63 per cent** often felt unsafe when out;
- **33 per cent** had been physically touched by people in public; and
- **12 per cent** had experienced physical violence.

I've experienced this myself – the laughter and mockery, the teasing, the name calling – midget, dwarf, half-pint, mutant, Mekon, goblin, short-arse, wee man. While on several occasions I have experienced direct harassment, I have never experienced physical violence. Others have been less lucky. It is for this reason that restricted growth people often prioritise having their own cars – because they are then insulated from the harassment they would receive when walking around or taking public transport.

While recorded hate crimes against disabled people have increased, this reflects, in part, increased awareness, better police response, and more reporting of incidents. There is a lack of good quality research on the topic. With data on adults, we immediately encounter the difficulty that it is often not clear whether the statistics are referring to disabled people who were victims of violence, or people who became disabled as a consequence of violence. To avoid this problem, a systematic review of the literature by colleagues at Liverpool John Moores University included only those studies of people with disabilities who had experienced violence in the last year. The review found that people with disabilities were 50 per cent more likely than non-disabled people to have experienced violence in the last year. This corresponds to 3 per cent of all disabled people. The raised risk was increased to four times more likely for people with mental health conditions, corresponding to nearly a quarter of people with mental health conditions experiencing violence in the last year. The overall lifetime risk of violence would have been much higher.

Since a new law in 1998, US Department of Justice has disaggregated statistics on disability violence in America. The 2008–2011 figures show that the average annual age-adjusted rate of serious violent victimisation for persons with disabilities (22 per thousand) was more than three times higher than that for non-disabled people (6 per thousand). The age-adjusted rate of simple assault for persons with disabilities (26 per thousand) was twice that for non-disabled people (13 per thousand). Men with disabilities suffered more violence in 2011 (42 per thousand) than women without disabilities (17 per thousand), but women with disabilities suffered the highest rate (53 per thousand). People with cognitive disabilities had by far the highest rates of victimisation. Serious violent victimisation increased for all disability groups between 2009 and 2011.

Eric Emerson and Alan Roulstone analysed the UK Life Opportunities Survey, which depends on self-report by disabled people. In this survey, it was people with mental health or behavioural difficulties who were most likely to experience violence, with a six-fold increased risk of violence and a ten times increased risk of hate crime. About 1 per cent of people with mobility impairments had experienced a disability-motivated hate crime in the previous year, rising to about 7 per cent of people with cognitive impairments.

The Liverpool John Moores team also conducted a systematic review of prevalence of violence against disabled children, and found that they were at 3.68 times the risk of non-disabled children, which corresponds to 26.7 per cent of disabled children having experienced violence in their lives. This risk was accentuated for children with learning difficulties or mental health conditions.

Why do disabled people seem to be disproportionately targeted? Disabled people may have vulnerabilities arising from impairment. The person with mobility impairment cannot run away; the blind or deaf person can less easily perceive danger; someone with a speech or language impairment cannot communicate what has happened to them; the physically frail person cannot defend themselves; a person with learning difficulties may be naïve and trusting or too open with information. People with learning difficulties, of all disabled people, seem the most likely to become victims of violence and abuse. However, other forms of vulnerability arise from the social context in which many disabled people are located. Historically, children and adults with disabilities in developed countries and former communist countries were more likely to be living in residential institutions. Rates of violence and abuse are often higher in residential settings. However, even in community settings, disabled children come into contact with many different adults: carers, taxi drivers, teachers, support workers, respite carers – and given that abusers are sometimes drawn to this area of work, there is likely to be a greater risk of abuse. In parts of Africa, one of the most hateful forms of abuse is the violence directed towards albino people, whose body parts are thought to be potent sources of magical power, and who are at risk of being dismembered or killed.

Since the welcome advent of community care policies, people with learning difficulties are less likely to be institutionalised – which takes them out of one situation of risk. Instead, they are likely to be living on their own or with one or two other people with learning difficulties in social housing, often in an area of social deprivation. People with learning difficulties may be isolated and lonely, and they may be highly visible and vulnerable to bored youth looking for 'fun' and possibly financial gain. If they or their family manage to complain to the authorities, there may be no follow-up on the complaint, or they may fear repercussions.

One response to the perception of vulnerability is protection policies. These can infringe the choices and freedoms of individuals. Paradoxically, over-protection may put people at risk, because people do not learn the skills to analyse interactions or cope with situations. In practice, vulnerability usually arises from the interaction of individual and contextual factors – the characteristics of the individual, and the context in which they find themselves. The answer is not to over-protect or segregate, but to empower, support, monitor and react quickly and effectively to any signs that things are going wrong.

Historically, UK police and criminal justice authorities have failed adequately to respond to violence and abuse directed at disabled people. Anti-social behaviour or intimidation may not be taken seriously by police. Police stations need to be physically accessible, to be better at listening to complaints and quicker and more effective at responding. There is growing awareness of these deficiencies of policing and action has been taken to offer a better service to disabled people. Victim support must begin with services which listen, believe and support people who have experienced violence, for example women with learning difficulties who have suffered intimate partner violence.

Across the world, various prevention and victim support measures have been tried. A Korean programme raised awareness of child abuse among parents of children with disabled children. Respite care reduced stress among parents of children with developmental disabilities. Various forms of behavioural skills training or decision-making have been tried for women with mild to moderate learning difficulties, which have produced improvements in knowledge and skills. British trainee police officers have undergone awareness training about learning difficulties. In South Africa, a sexual assault victim empowerment programme led to victims with learning difficulties achieving the same conviction rate against their attackers as non-disabled women. In countries such as Tanzania, Kenya and Uganda, education and awareness can improve traditional attitudes towards albino people and reduce the incidence of violence.

CONCLUSION

This chapter has looked at different facets of impairment and disability across the life course, from childhood to old age. Shared experiences, like becoming disabled, rehabilitation, independent living and violence and abuse, may be experienced at any age. There is growing research evidence about these different aspects of life as a disabled person. In some areas – such as preventing and responding to violence – raised awareness has driven an improved response. In other areas – such as independent living and social care – funding cuts in the UK and other developed countries have diminished opportunities and impact quality of life.

FURTHER READING

Gillian Parker. 1993. *With this Body: caring and disability within marriage.* Buckingham: Open University Press.

Mark Priestley. 2003. *Disability: a life course approach.* Cambridge: Polity.

Katharine Quarmby. 2011. *Scapegoat: why we are failing disabled people.* London: Portobello Books.

Tom Shakespeare, Kath Gillespie-Sells and Dominic Davies. 1996. *The Sexual Politics of Disability: untold desires.* London: Cassell.

Steve Silberman. 2014. *Neurotribes: the legacy of autism and the future of neurodiversity.* New York: Avery.

Andrew Sullivan. 2012. *Far From the Tree: parents, children and the search for identity.* New York: Scribner.

DISABLING BARRIERS

In Chapter 1, we encountered the social model of disability – the idea that people are disabled by society, rather than by their bodies. It's time to look more closely at how this operates. In this chapter, I want to explore further the concept of disabling barriers, concentrating on three dimensions: the physical and information environment; the role of negative attitudes; and the possibilities of equal opportunities in employment. Putting three very different phenomena in the same chapter may seem random. But in each case, failures by society render many disabled people excluded, damaged or disadvantaged. In each case, the problem is fundamentally one of the attitudes and behaviours of the non-disabled world. Even when barriers derive from a physical building, transport system or technology, it has been the choice of some person to construct them in an enabling or disabling way, to offer supportive help or to neglect a disabled user. These three dimensions do not exhaust the many ways in which people with impairments are disabled by society, but to me they seem the most pressing examples of how barriers so deeply affect people's lives and opportunities.

ENVIRONMENTAL BARRIERS

When there is no transport and the school is miles away, or when it has no accessible toilet, or when the hospital or university has steps, then disabled people are effectively excluded. I remember the wheelchair user I met in Egypt, who told me that she had the choice of either drinking water or getting an education, because the local school had no toilet that was accessible to her. At some risk to her health, and with help from school friends carrying her wheelchair upstairs, she completed her education, then got her degree, then a PhD, and ended up in Parliament. I remember the young polio survivor I met in Zambia. Proudly, he told me that he was the only member of his family who had finished school. I looked at the crutches he used to walk with, and thought of the dusty, rocky, pot-holed roads I had seen in Africa. He then explained that it had taken him three hours, morning and after-noon, to get to school and back. It is the rare child who is not defeated by such obstacles.

As these stories show, barrier-free buildings and transport are important not just in themselves, but also because they enable people to access other public goods, such as education, health and employment opportunities. But accessibility is not just a matter of ramps and toilets. It also depends on information and signage, for people with sensory impairments. Another dimension is the positive attitudes, so that people with the whole range of impair-ments are welcomed. The alterations that are required to ensure that disabled people enjoy a barrier-free environment are not usually costly. But these changes require political commitment, accessibility guidelines, and a willingness to enforce the law.

In the wake of the 2012 Olympic and Paralympic Games in London, the most accessible Games ever, the Built Environment Professional Education Project was undertaken in the UK to promote inclusive design. Together with widespread awareness raising, some progress was achieved in influencing the teaching of architecture and related disciplines. The British Institute of Facil-ities Management, the Chartered Institute of Architectural Technologists and the Royal Town Planning Institute all intro-duced accessibility and inclusion into the professional standards they require of students. Other professional bodies are also likely to add these competencies into training requirements. When architecture professionals truly understand what is required to achieve access, then perhaps people will be less excluded.

TRANSPORT FOR ALL?

The disability rights dream is for barrier-free transport, where no special provision is needed, and where, regardless of sight, hearing, mobility or other differences, the disabled person can use the same bus, tram or train. In some settings, this is a reality. In Curitiba, a city in eastern Brazil, the bus rapid transport system is designed to be accessible to all. It makes commuting easier for everyone, and presents no barriers to disabled people. In London, the new stretch of the Jubilee line is accessible between Westminster and Stratford stations, and so is the Docklands Light Railway. Around the world, there are a few other examples, such as low-floor buses which can be more easily accessed by ambulant disabled people. But even accessible public transport still does not always have accessible information: visually impaired disability advocate Graeme Innes fought a long legal battle to ensure that his local Sydney light rail transport include audible announcements of each stop, rather than just an illuminated display.

After decades of campaigning and with the aid of legislative changes, many more mainstream transport options have become accessible, with a degree of assistance. The London black cab is designed to be accessible by ramp – if the driver is willing to help. Staff on the Tokyo subway are able to provide access ramps for disabled passengers to board the trains. Subways in cities such as Barcelona and Delhi and Beijing are also accessible. With a day's notice in advance, the companies that run Britain's railways will provide ramps and reserve wheelchair spaces for disabled people. The buses in London or New York or Paris are fitted with mechanical ramps: when they are operational, when the bus driver is willing, and when the bus is not congested, the wheelchair user can board. In the UK, nearly 90 per cent of buses now have low floor wheelchair access. Almost all airports are willing to accept disabled passengers if they book assistance in advance. Aisle chairs and bigger bathrooms make the flying experience easier. But plane travel is much easier for people who have some residual mobility, or who are not very tall or heavy, than for people who have high support needs, or who are heavy, when it is hard for them to be lifted in and out of seats.

All of these transport solutions depend on efficient and courteous non-disabled people who are available and willing to help, something which cannot always be taken for granted. Many of these adaptations need booking in advance. A truly accessible world would be one where disabled people could turn up, secure in the knowledge that they would be accommodated. In all cases, the provision of information – now usually accessed mainly on the internet – enables disabled people to understand whether there is level access, or whether ramps or other assistance are needed.

But the majority of the world's transport is not accessible to disabled people. For example, the *matatu* minibuses or *boda-boda* motorcycles which transport people around African cities are not accessible to most disabled people. Where there are buses in developing countries, these are often former school buses donated from the United States, or other traditional models which do not have ramps or spaces or easy access for people with mobility impairments. In many of the world's cities, ordinary saloon taxis present barriers to disabled people who cannot transfer out of their wheelchair, or who have power chairs. The vast majority of London's Tube system is inaccessible to anyone with mobility impairment. A fifth of UK disabled people still report difficulties in accessing transport.

As well as public transport, roads and road crossings are also issues for people with mobility or sight difficulties in developing countries. Multi-lane highways with continuously moving traffic, which are the everyday reality in cities like Cairo or Delhi or Kampala or Manila, are very difficult for anyone to cross. For people with disabilities they provide an added burden, even a risk to life. The absence of a flat and even sidewalk offers further challenges to someone who relies on a wheelchair, or crutches, or cannot see obstacles. This makes independent travel very difficult for disabled people, unless they have assistance.

Whether in a high-, low- or middle-income country, transport access is not just important in itself. It also underpins access to health, education and employment, all vital aspects of life. When disabled people cannot travel, they cannot take part in society. Solutions are possible, but they require commitment, planning and some investment. They should be a priority.

BUILDING IT RIGHT FROM THE START

Making buildings accessible is not hard. Wide doors, level access, elevators, spacious public toilets, clear signage all mean that people with a range of impairments can easily enter and move about. The additional cost of making a public building accessible is minimal. This was proved during the design stage of the Durban International Convention Centre in South Africa. The original plans lacked accessibility. This was discovered, and thanks to the participation of disabled people, a revised plan was developed by the architects. The additional costs were less than 1 per cent of the total build cost.

It is harder and more costly to retrofit a building which was constructed in a previous century, or else was designed by an architect who showed disregard for the diversity of the population. Often, the accessible entrance is round the back of the building, because the main entrance is dominated by an imposing but impractical flight of steps. Sometimes, the disabled visitor has to enter via the kitchen area. But inspired architects have shown that even in an historic building, it is possible to achieve good access without damaging the fabric or harming the special feeling of an ancient space.

Aside from schools and hospitals, most public buildings are less indispensable to the good life, although barriers send the message that disabled people are second class citizens. I remember when I lived in Geneva going to see an advertised exhibition at the local ethnographic museum, only to find it was upstairs and there was no lift: as a result, I felt dismayed and excluded. But housing is essential for everyone. In the era of Victorian terraces and bulky wheelchairs, living in the community was very difficult for many British disabled people. The development of small, lightweight wheelchairs revolutionised access. The post-war construction of bungalows, and also new social housing, with lifts and ramps, also offered new options to disabled people leaving residential institutions in the 1970s and 1980s. Today, new building standards, such as the Lifetime Homes concept, which includes features such as level access and wide doors, mean that there is more chance of disabled and older people being able to use ordinary housing stock, rather than having to invest in expensive retro-fitting. But still, despite improvements, UK surveys show that, 1 in 3 households with a disabled person still live in non-decent accommodation, and 1 in 5 disabled people requiring adaptations to their home believe that their accommodation is not suitable.

Housing is not just a matter of physical fabric; it is also about policy. In the UK, the Thatcherite policy of selling off council houses meant that ground-floor flats with gardens were often the first to go – and these were usually the most accessible dwellings. After 2010, the Coalition and then successive Conservative governments' policy of the 'under occupancy penalty', better known as the 'bedroom tax', meant that social housing tenants were penalised for having more bedrooms than residents. But disabled people often require this extra space, either for equipment – such as wheelchairs or hoists – or else for sleep-in personal assistants. Thus disabled people ended up being victimised by this provision. Overall, the sale of council houses, and limited new builds, means that it has been difficult for disabled people to find appropriate accommodation. Often, people with learning diffi-culties have been placed in flats in areas of social deprivation, where they have sometimes been at risk of hate crime.

In low-income settings, housing is often over-crowded. Inac-cessible latrines or squat toilets also disadvantage many people. These problems of housing are even more difficult in informal settlements. Even if people have access to a wheelchair, uneven surfaces and rocky terrains makes access difficult for disabled people with mobility or sight difficulties, while mud is a hazard when it rains. Yet solutions can be found. For example, in Sri Lanka after the tsunami of December 2004, low-income housing together with accessible latrines were constructed for villagers in coastal communities.

Housing difficulties can keep disabled people stuck in one place, perhaps with parents or a partner that they need to separate from, or isolated from their friends. The lack of accessible accommodation means that it is difficult for disabled people to move somewhere else for employment. It is also means that older people, when they become disabled, often cannot move out of hospital and back home. People with mobility difficulties sometimes have to move into old people's homes or other congregate living, purely because their own homes are not accessible. This makes it a priority to ensure that new housing includes accessible, affordable living spaces, and these are reserved for people who need them.

INFORMATION AND COMMUNICATION TECHNOLOGIES

In the twenty-first century, accessible environments refer to ICT and the online world, as well as to physical settings. ICT has the potential to liberate people, or further to exclude them. For example, JAWS screen reader software means that people with visual impairment can operate computers and read websites and electronic books. However, JAWS works best for languages like English and French, rather than for rarer local languages. Deaf people can communicate with each other by text or can sign together using Skype. People on the autistic spectrum, who may find face to face interaction difficult, may be able to connect with people at a distance through email and web. But in each case, the disabled person first has to be able to buy a computer and any necessary software ($1,000 for JAWS), and pay for internet access. In 2011, 61 per cent of UK disabled people lived in households with internet access, compared with 86 per cent of non-disabled people. Similarly, smartphones enable people with sensory impairments to stay connected, if they can afford them: Android and iPhone devices come with built-in screen-readers.

These information and communication technologies are essential for people with sensory impairment to participate in school, as well as in the workplace, so long as they can access them. Ensuring that pupils and students with sensory impairments have teaching materials appropriate to them, or human readers to enable them to access necessary texts, has been a struggle, particularly in developing countries.

Developments in ICT can either include or exclude disabled people. Braille printers have made text accessible. E-books are another step forward; touch screens on a phone or tablet are a step back. But the Flash multi-media platform has made web browsing difficult. People with dexterity limitations or tremors may find touch screens or mouse control difficult. Because platforms and programmes are continually being developed and being upgraded, accessibility plug-ins may be superseded and adaptations may need to be made from scratch each time. Compatibility of company intranets with adaptive technologies is often a problem. Even online job application systems may present barriers for people with visual or dexterity limitations.

Websites can be designed to be accessible to all, so that a screen reader can communicate the contents to a visually impaired user. But this requires the designer to conform to the Web Content Accessibility Guidelines (WCAG). Tables or forms on webpages are a common problem. Visual images on webpages require meta-tags, so that the visually impaired user receives a text description of what the image contains, when they roll their mouse over it. In the UK, websites are legally obliged to be accessible to visually impaired users, but this is rarely enforced.

For deaf people, the key technology is closed captioning of broadcast television and online video. Progress had been made with live broadcast and broadcasts of pre-recorded material. However, online video and video-on-demand has not been captioned to the same degree. Closed captioning is available on YouTube, but only if the person who creates or uploads the video clip adds it.

Different countries have different laws and different requirements. For a long time, the limited national copyright exemptions to allow visually impaired readers to get electronic copies of books prevented these accessible texts crossing borders. The 2013 Marrakesh Treaty to Facilitate Access to Published Works by Visually Impaired Persons and Persons with Print Disabilities (MVT for short) has been a huge step forward, as it overcame these intellectual property problems.

Developments in technology change the world for disabled and deaf users, sometimes for better, sometimes for worse. For example, the past, every town had a Deaf Club, where sign language users would meet on the same night of the week to meet other people, find out what was going on locally and make plans. In the era of skype and smartphones, Deaf people can stay connected without physically meeting. Partly as a result, many Deaf Clubs are closing down or under threat.

As with physical access barriers, the problems of ICT access are about human choices, not technological limitations. In every instance, a solution can be found, if people are willing to ensure that their sites or handsets or broadcasts are accessible to all. If people forget or ignore disabled users, then the outcome will be discriminatory barriers. In an age dominated by new media and communication, being excluded from ICT will reinforce traditional barriers to work and society.

ATTITUDES

Attitudes are central to the disability experience. When policy-makers, architects, engineers and designers have the right attitudes, they are more likely to commission or construct accessible facilities. Within environments – hospitals and schools and workplaces and leisure facilities – non-disabled people can make people feel welcome and included when they have the right attitudes. Supportive attitudes make access easier – while negative attitudes create barriers in themselves. It makes no difference if the hospital is accessible, when the pregnant disabled woman faces incredulous laughter from the health workers when she arrives at the maternity ward, a story I heard in Mali. The Deaf woman I met in Uganda reported that in her village, everyone said her impairment was the result of witchcraft. 'This daughter will never amount to anything', they told her parents. She had fought against such negative attitudes, done very well in school despite not being able to hear the teacher, and ended up as an education professional, developing curricula for schools.

In the UK, attitude surveys show that negative attitudes are being slowly replaced with more accepting attitudes. This may be to do with higher levels of education and acceptance more generally. It may be to do with greater visibility of disabled achievers in the media – including the effect of televising the Paralympic games. Familiarity with almost anything makes it less alarming and more accepted.

Yet these advances are precarious. Media and government discourse around welfare benefits can result in negativity towards claimants. The public makes a distinction between the 'genuine' disabled people, who are entitled to support, and 'scroungers' who are defrauding the system or who do not have 'genuine' impairments, and who should be punished. Glasgow Media Group and Strathclyde Centre for Disability Research have analysed how negative language and stories in the press contribute towards prejudice.

For example, one British disabled man told me how, when he was about to get into his adapted vehicle, a passing mother with her child in a pushchair retorted 'I paid for that car', suggesting resentment about Personal Independence Payments and the Motability scheme. Only afterwards did the disabled person think that he might equally have replied 'I paid for that baby', referring to the Child Benefit scheme. In a period where real wages are frozen and people's benefits are under threat, and when the print media whip up indignation against immigrants and benefit cheats, it is unsurprising that negative attitudes increase as a result.

Negative images and attitudes about disability derive from a range of stereotypes. Sometimes, disability is conceptualised in terms of dependency and disease – the pathetic 'Tiny Tim' cripple of Charles Dickens, or the Victorian children's story. Traditionally, charity advertising used similar images, particularly of children, to generate pity in the viewer, and raise money for the needy. Disability activists have long objected to these patronising and negative images, which reinforce negative thinking about disability.

Sometimes, disability is seen as threatening – literally sinister, deriving from the Latin *sinestra*, referring to left-handed people. From Shakespeare's Richard III to the deformed villains of legend this is clearly a very negative stereotype. Physical difference or disfigurement connotes moral twistedness also. Baddies like Long John Silver or Captain Hook or more recently the villains of the James Bond films, generate fear and hostility from non-disabled viewers. They are portrayed as bitter and villainous, often, because they have not come to terms with their impairment. Again, these associate disability with negativity.

Finally, there is a distorted 'super crip' idea, referring to the disabled person who has overcome his or her difficulties and triumphed over them. He or she is not bitter, not twisted, just determined. Sometimes the disabled person, like the autistic hero of the film *Rain Man*, has compensatory abilities. These tropes even influence the ways in which Professor Stephen Hawking is described, or the many media stories about people who have overcome the odds, including war veterans like Douglas Bader, or those Paralympic champions, particularly ex-service people.

The late Australian comedienne and writer Stella Young parodied patronising attitudes about disability when she talked about 'inspiration porn'. She was referring to the tendency to celebrate even very minor achievements by disabled people, and to see the ordinary lives of people with significant impairment as being somehow marvellous or, to use a common but hated term, 'plucky'. The disabled child gets an award, simply for turning up to school or performing in a concert. A common trope is to say 'if this disabled person overcame the odds, then you too can be inspired to overcome your own troubles'. But as Stella said, disabled people are not here to teach non-disabled people lessons about grit and determination.

Of course, disabled people want to be treated like everyone else. We are more like everyone else than we are different. We are typically complex human beings, capable of brilliance and failure, kindness and cruelty. Disability does not determine character, although it may influence us. Many people have indeed overcome obstacles, but often people minimise any difficulties, because they have got used to them. If barriers are just part of their life, it's strange to them when other people express admiration or concern or amazement at what they take for granted. Sometimes non-disabled people imagine what it must be like to be disabled, but their imagination gets it wrong. They feel that they could not cope, without a major sense, for example, and therefore think of disabled people as super-heroic when they seem to manage fine.

Because non-disabled people are often anxious about interacting with someone with a visible impairment, or have false beliefs about disability, then there is pressure on the disabled person to manage the interaction in order to overcome the stigma, to use the terminology of Erving Goffman. The disabled person has to set the non-disabled person at their ease, if they are to have a smooth dialogue with them. People who are born with an impairment often develop great communication skills, or have a good sense of humour, as an adaptive response. In order for interactions to go well, they have to take responsibility, make a joke, and thus demonstrate that all is well, and there is no need for the non-disabled person to be anxious.

Whereas being patronised is irritating, and it may be exhausting to manage other people's unease, negative attitudes can impact more oppressively when they fuel bullying or hostility, as discussed in the previous chapter. For example, disabled people are 50 per cent more likely than non-disabled people to experience unfairness, discrimination, bullying or harassment at work. Disabled people are also at risk when they live in the community. Bullying, abuse and violence generate fear and create harm for disabled people, sometimes resulting in death. Even disabled people who have not experienced these extreme attitudes live in fear, and change their routines to avoid places which they perceive as risky.

DISCRIMINATION IN EMPLOYMENT

According to the UK Labour Force Survey, roughly 12 per cent of working-age people are defined as having a disability – in other words, an impairment which substantially and adversely affects amount and/or type of work, as well as activities of daily living. Although only 9 per cent of disabled people of working age have never had a job, disabled people are significantly disadvantaged in the area of employment. This is partly to do with the consequences of a disabling health condition. One third of disabled people in work, and two-thirds of disabled people out of work, say their health condition impacts their ability to work. For example, some disabled people will have lower productivity than non-disabled people. Flexible working – such as changes to working hours, work schedules, tasks, environments – can make it easier for a disabled person to work. But some disabled people are so limited by their impairment – mental or physical – that they cannot do any work at all.

But employment disadvantage is also to do with social factors. Many disabled young people leave school with no or inferior qualifications, and they are less likely to transition to tertiary education. People can face discrimination in getting a job if they have a disability, and keeping a job if they become disabled. Negative attitudes or low expectations from careers advisors or recruitment officers play a gate-keeping role, steering people away from the careers that they dream of. Employers may regard disabled people as too costly or unreliable. Access barriers mean that transport to a workplace and access within a workplace may be limited, as well as issues of communication to overcome, for example getting support for sign language interpreters.

As a result of these intrinsic and extrinsic factors, there is still a large gap in the UK employment rate. In 2012, 46.3 per cent of working-age disabled people were in employment compared with 76.4 per cent of working-age non-disabled people. The disability employment gap (between employment of disabled and non-disabled people) remains at about 30 per cent, but has reduced by 10 percentage points over the last 14 years. Among the most disadvantaged are people with mental health conditions, whose employment rate is less than 15 per cent, and people with learning difficulties, only 6 per cent of whom are employed. In 2015, the American Bureau of Labour Statistics reported that 26.9 per cent of adults with disabilities of working age were employed, as compared with 72.2 per cent of individuals without disabilities. This rate was even lower for adults with learning difficulties. Thirty-two per cent of disabled workers were in part time jobs, compared with 18 per cent of workers without a disability. The unemployment rate for disabled people was 10.7 per cent, compared with 5.1 per cent for non-disabled people.

Research by the Higher Education Funding Council for England (HEFCE) in 2015 finds that 40 months after leaving higher education, the employment rate for graduates with no known disability was 96.6 per cent; 77.8 per cent were working in a professional or managerial role. However, the employment rate for those who had declared a disability, but did not receive Disabled Students' Allowance was slightly lower, at 94.8 per cent; 73.8 per cent were working in a professional or managerial role. Employment for those who did receive DSA was lower still at 93.7 per cent, with 73.1 per cent working in a professional or managerial role. While substantially better than the average employment rate of disabled people (46.3 per cent), this shows that disabled graduate employment remains lower than that of non-disabled people, and 5.1 per cent lower for professional or managerial roles.

What can be done about these barriers in the labour market? The disability employment gap is a persistent problem in most developed economies. The cause appears to be a combination of employer discrimination, low educational achievement, and lower productivity. Some disabled people even anticipate barriers and do not attempt to find work, thus disengaging from the labour market.

Two traditional responses have been sheltered employment and disability quotas. Sheltered employment is the segregated solution, setting up factories or other businesses which cater particularly for disabled workers: these were the chief response to the increased numbers of disabled people trying to enter the labour market after the Second World War. However, as the economy has changed, sheltered employment has required higher and higher subsidies. The hope that disabled workers would move out of sheltered employment into the open labour market has never been realised. In recent years, the UK government has withdrawn subsidy from Remploy, the main provider of sheltered employment, and factories have closed, making disabled people redundant. By contrast, Switzerland still maintains sheltered workshops and as a consequence reports a high level of disabled employment. As an alternative to sheltered employment, supported employment is about enabling individuals to gain employment in the open market. This is now more favoured, with a particular emphasis on 'place and train' approaches, where individuals get assistance on the job, rather than training before they apply for jobs. Working to change employer attitudes, as with the Ntiro Project for Supported and Inclusive Employment in South Africa, maximises the chances of success.

In the post-war period, some countries have tried an employment quota for disabled people, levying a fine on companies that did not comply. For example, in the UK, the 1944 Disabled Persons (Employment) Act mandated a 3 per cent quota of registered disabled people. But this was ineffectual. Many employers obtained exemption certificates. Others just ignored the law – and could do so with impunity, because so few people were prosecuted. In the end, people stopped registering as disabled, and eventually the evidence even showed that registered disabled people were more likely to be unemployed as those who were not registered. There is a similar story from Brazil, where employers would rather pay the financial penalty, or give disabled people token employment, than implement the quota. In other countries, such as Germany and Japan, quotas may have been more successful. However, in signalling that disabled people cannot compete in the labour market and need special protection, the quota approach is perhaps counter-productive to efforts to change negative attitudes about disability.

Many programmes to get people into work, such as the US Ticket to Work employment programme, have been ineffective. In the UK, the Labour government from 1997 promoted a series of New Deal programmes, under the mantra of 'work for those who can, security for those who cannot'. But these Pathways to Work initiatives mainly focused on the unemployed individual ('supply side'), rather than the potential employer ('demand side'). For example, providing vocational training, health advice, financial incentives/penalties. In low-income countries, there are many examples of vocational training schemes. Traditionally, craft skills such as tailoring and shoe-making were popular. With mass production of cheap shoes and clothes, training to be a craftsperson seems a less sensible strategy, and consequently there is an emphasis on IT skills. It is very important to provide training relevant to the local market demand.

One response, the UK Access to Work scheme has covered many of the costs associated with employing disabled people, relieving the employer of the burden. This benefit has been very successful in helping disabled people enter the workplace, for example covering the additional costs of employment for disabled people, such as travel to work, costs of personal assistants at work, costs of sign language interpreters, costs of assistive technologies. However, in the era of austerity, there have been cuts to entitlements which risk excluding people from the workforce, particularly Deaf people who are reliant on sign language interpreters.

A key structural change, which should in principle promote employment, is anti-discrimination legislation. But law may sometimes have paradoxical effects. The 1990 Americans with Disabilities Act was associated with a decrease in employment for disabled Americans, because it was perceived to increase costs for employers, and make it more difficult to get rid of disabled work-ers. More positively, the legal concept of 'reasonable accommodation' – or 'reasonable adjustment' in the UK – is an important benchmark. It signals that employers – or other duty-bearers – must take reasonable steps to improve accessibility or accommodate individual needs. This might include making changes to workspaces or to work schedules, or providing tech-nologies. The Convention on the Rights of Persons with Disabilities and some national laws state that 'denial of reasonable accommodation constitutes discrimination'. Whereas employers fear that making reasonable accommodation will be very costly, the majority of adjustments are cost-free or less than $1,000. In the UK, the Equality Act 2010 makes it legal to discriminate positively in favour of a disabled applicant – the only area in which positive discrimination is permitted. However, legislation mostly relies on individuals resorting to litigation when they perceive themselves to be victims of discrimination, which is complex and costly to carry through to success.

Within work, disabled people can experience a similar glass ceiling to other disadvantaged groups: they are overrepresented in lower occupational roles, and much less likely to be in managerial and professional roles. This may be partly due to discrimination and partly due to poor educational achievement. My research team found that our restricted growth respondents had educa-tional qualifications equivalent to or better than their non-disabled peers. However, we found that they had been discouraged from considering better careers, because of low expectations from others. They had also tended to stick in junior roles, which they were performing well in, and where they were accepted, rather than risk losing what they had gained by striving to be promoted to a more senior role. These fears may have some justification, given the surveys that have shown that disabled people are 50 per cent more likely to have suffered unfairness, discrimination, bullying or harassment at work compared with non-disabled people.

In the UK, disabled people are 14 per cent more likely to work part time than non-disabled people. Disabled people are far more likely to retire early than non-disabled people, as we found in our restricted growth study and Nicholas Watson found in a small research study he conducted with older people with cerebral palsy. These pay disparities are found throughout the developed world. Across 27 industrialised economies, the pay gap between disabled and non-disabled people averaged 15 per cent. These disparities can also be found in developing countries.

All this means that the incomes of disabled people are likely to be lower: in the UK, 30 per cent earn less than the living wage, according to the Equality and Human Rights Commission, as compared with 26 per cent of non-disabled people. In addition, many disabled people are faced with extra costs as a result of their health condition or the social barriers. The effect of unemployment and underemployment plus extra costs is increased poverty among disabled people, and greater dependency on government welfare payments: in the UK, 'Incapacity Benefit', now called 'Employment Support Allowance'; in the US, 'Social Security Disability Insurance' or 'Supplemental Security Income'. In the UK at the time of writing, 19 per cent of families with one or more disabled members live in relative poverty, before housing costs, compared with 15 per cent of families with no disabled members; 21 per cent of children in families with a disabled member are in poverty, compared with 16 per cent of children in families with no disabled members. Many people still do not claim benefits to which they may be entitled, and specialist advice and support is required to gain access to entitlements, particularly as many people are not successful in being awarded benefits unless they appeal after the initial rejection of their applications. Worldwide, a survey of 27 high-income countries found that disabled people were more likely to live under the poverty threshold in 24 of those countries. A study in low- and middle-income countries found significantly worse economic well-being in 14 out of 15 countries. Over time, these disparities in income are not improving. This level of poverty and economic exclusion is not just harmful to individuals: it also harms economies, in terms of wasted human capital, more people requiring social assistance, fewer people paying tax.

In recent decades, as the numbers of people claiming disability benefits have increased, governments have made renewed efforts to get disabled people into work and off benefit rolls. These have been combinations of 'sticks' – reducing the level of payments, making benefits harder to get, increased conditionality (insisting that claimants comply with reporting or job application requirements) – and 'carrots' – support with additional costs of employment, job counselling, supported employment and other measures. A key transition point has been where short-term sickness absence turns into long-term disability, which makes it harder and harder to get back into the labour market. Trying to prevent this transition, and trying to stop young disabled people going straight onto benefits rather than entering the labour market, have been priorities for governments seeking to reduce the cost of welfare.

In the UK, Labour introduced, and the subsequent Coalition government amplified, the role of the Work Capability Assessment, as a gateway to the Employment Support Allowance benefit. Whereas before, a disabled person was assessed in terms of their likelihood of finding a job, after the 'reforms', disabled people were assessed in terms of their theoretical ability to work. This difference meant that fewer people were allocated the welfare benefit. Disabled people are assessed either as being unable to work and put into a 'support' group, or as being able to do some form of work, where they are placed into a 'work-related activity' group, and steered towards employment opportunities. If they do not comply, the level of benefit is reduced. These sanctions, on people who are already in poverty, can have drastic effects, particularly on people with mental health problems. Evidence shows that rates of mental health treatment and rates of suicide are higher in areas where there have been more ESA reassessments. Australian changes to the Disability Support Pension from 2006 are along similar lines to those in Britain. But punitive measures do not seem a fair or effective response to people who are struggling to find work.

In the UK, the Business Disability Forum (formerly the Employers Forum on Disability) has been using persuasion and education tactics for twenty years. It has now recruited nearly 400 employers to its programme. By working with big companies, who want to be seen as progressive, and are prepared to take the risk of offering disabled people roles, this agency has managed to have some impact by equipping employers with appropriate skills and advising on best practice. The approach has been to stress the business case – that disabled people make very good employees – rather than to appeal to the soft heart of employers. The same model has been tried in other countries, including Argentina, Brazil, Spain, Sri Lanka and Vietnam.

In developing countries, disabled people access livelihood opportunities in the informal sector, as self-employed craftspeople, shopkeepers and farmers. Community-based rehabilitation (CBR) stresses access to livelihood, which often means small scale enterprises. However, access to credit is a big barrier. Research by the NGO Handicap International in seven developing countries found that less than 1 per cent of microfinance customers were known to have disabilities. In my research in Africa, I have also interviewed dozens of disabled people who overcame barriers to complete schooling and get a job as a teacher or a civil servant or working for a voluntary organisation or disabled people's organisation. Disabled people face ignorance and discrimination in all fields, and have to work twice as hard to overcome these attitudinal barriers and achieve success. But as low- and middle-income countries transition to more developed economies, the risk is that disabled people will be excluded from livelihood opportunities, because informal work gives way to formal employment.

Given that one-third of people in work and two thirds of disabled people out of work are limited in the type or amount of work they can do, according to UK estimates, any efforts to enable disabled people to win employment have to take account of these limitations. The OECD's 2009 *Sickness, Disability and Work* report suggests that a culture of inclusion is required, an approach based on capacity not incapacity, involving structural reforms, not just short-term strategies. Ensuring that young people with disabilities in education make a successful transition to employment is crucial, but many efforts in this area have been ineffective. Role models help. So do imaginative forms of supported employment, such as social firms, which compete in the market but have social goals, such as having learning disabled or mentally ill people working alongside non-disabled people. More people in Britain are employed than ever before, albeit often in low paid or insecure jobs. On the one hand, this means that disabled workers will be desirable, to fill employment gaps –

especially after Britain leaves the European Union. But disabled people currently receiving welfare benefits will not want to risk their status by trying to work, if the insecurity of employment means they might later lose their job. It is important to give disabled people security, so that they know their additional costs will be met, and that they can try out work without threatening their security.

CONCLUSION

Barriers to the equal participation of disabled people, particularly access and attitudes, are perennial problems that hold back full equality. At least there is growing awareness of the issue. As of 2016, the Women and Equalities Committee of the UK House of Commons has launched an inquiry into accessibility of buildings, private spaces and homes. The UK Police are taking hate crime and violence against disabled people more seriously. The UK Government has pledged to reduce the disability employment gap, and has made some progress. At the international level, the Committee on the Rights of Persons with Disabilities are interrogating governments about what they are doing to promote awareness (Article 8), access (Article 9) and employment (Article 27). Understanding that these are human rights issues of the gravest importance makes it more likely that they will be treated with the seriousness that they deserve.

FURTHER READING

Jody Heymann, Michael Ashley Stein and Gonzalo Moreno, editors. 2014. *Disability and Equity at Work*. Oxford: Oxford University Press.

Higher Education Funding Council for England. 2015. *Differences in Employment Outcomes: equality and diversity characteristics*. Bristol: Higher Education Funding Council for England.

Alan Roulstone and Colin Barnes, editors. 2005. *Working Futures? Disabled people, policy and social inclusion*. Bristol: Policy Press.

World Health Organization and World Bank. 2011. *World Report on Disability*. Geneva: World Health Organization.

HEALTH AND SOCIAL CARE

INTRODUCTION

In this chapter, I want to give an overview of issues concerning access to health for disabled people. The chapter will explore prevention, disabled people's health needs, access to mainstream health and rehabilitation, and then the specialist provision for people with learning difficulties and people with mental health conditions. In Article 25, Health, and Article 26, Rehabilitation, the Convention on the Rights of Persons with Disabilities emphasises that access to good quality healthcare is a human rights issue. Disability is more than a health issue – it is a social and economic issue. But disabled people do have health needs, as I will explore below. Unless basic health needs are met, then children and adults with disabilities cannot enjoy their other rights – to attend school, to participate in the community, to get a job. Rehabilitation interventions such as an appropriate wheelchair or speech and language therapy can make the difference between being included, and being left on the margins. Yet across the world, disabled people lack access to health and rehabilitation services. They face barriers and prejudice, or poorer quality healthcare. This means their health outcomes are worse – not as a result of their underlying impairments, but because of failures of general healthcare.

That is why it is so important for health professionals and researchers to understand the disability rights agenda and disability studies approach. At the same time, disability rights advocates have to acknowledge the value of medical and rehabilitation interventions, which in the past they have often rejected as being normalising or inappropriate. In particular, professionals need to adopt the human rights principles of respect, dignity, equality and non-discrimination in their interactions with disabled people. The best services in the world risk leaving patients and clients with disabilities alienated and bruised if they are not delivered with the appropriate communication skills and high ethical standards of care, which begin with listening to the individual.

PREVENTION

For disability rights activists, prevention of health conditions leading to disability can be a controversial topic. Because disability is increasingly regarded as a matter of equal opportunities, not medical problems, it could appear inconsistent to try and prevent people becoming disabled. Certainly, public health messages can be disparaging to disabled people, for example where they portray disability as a tragedy or in terms of dependency. Sensitivity is required to promote disability rights and equality, alongside reducing the incidence of preventable impairment. Because disability is a complex and multi-factorial phenomenon, efforts need to be made to reduce disabling barriers, as well as to reduce the incidence of disabling impairment or illnesses. A multi-faceted approach is needed.

Prenatal screening is a topic which can raise concerns (see Chapter 7 and appendix). Provision of balanced information, support, and informed consent should help reduce any negative dimensions of screening. Other preventive measures in the pre-conception period include reduction of hazardous factors in the environment (such as drugs, chemical exposures and industrial radiation), and dietary supplementation. In some countries, for example Canada, folate is added to flour, leading to a halving of the number of pregnancies affected by neural tube defects such as spina bifida. To take another example, fetal alcohol syndrome is associated with learning disabilities, and alcohol misuse can potentially be reduced through measures such as alcohol pricing and maternal education.

In most developed countries, every child is screened at birth with a heel prick, followed by analysis of bloods. This neonatal screening can identify cases of phenylketonuria (PKU), leading to dietary modification to ensure that learning disability does not result, as well as cystic fibrosis and sickle cell disease, so the relevant treatment can begin early. Infant screening can also identify hearing loss early, so that supportive measures can be put in place to prevent developmental delay.

Focusing on one particular impairment, spinal cord injury, shows how effective action can reduce the incidence of disabling conditions. The major traumatic causes of spinal cord injury (SCI) are road traffic injury and falls. In some parts of the world, violence is a third major cause: for example, nearly two-fifths of all SCI in sub Saharan Africa results from violence; in USA, one in eight cases of SCI is the results of gun violence. Sports and recreational injuries are another cause of spinal cord injury, and also implicated in head injury. Incidence can be reduced, for example by safe traffic systems, by occupational safety, by gun control, and by programmes to increase awareness and change rules around sports such as rugby and diving. In the developing world, enabling people to use wheelbarrows rather than carrying heavy loads on the head would reduce the incidence of cervical spinal injury. Main causes of non-traumatic SCI are tuberculosis, HIV and cancers. Here too, prevention interventions can reduce the incidence of SCI.

To take another example, visual impairment, WHO estimated in 2010 that 285 million people were visually impaired, of whom 39 million were blind. Eighty per cent of this visual impairment is avoidable. A third of visual impairment is caused by cataracts, for which basic surgery is effective. Trachoma is the leading infective cause of blindness, affecting 8 million people, followed by river blindness (onchocerciasis). The prevalence and impact of trachoma can be reduced by a combination of environmental improvements, hygiene, antibiotics and surgery in the advanced stages of the disease. River blindness can be treated by Ivermectin, which kills the parasite responsible. International NGOs such as

Light for the World and Sightsavers run campaigns to raise money to do this vital ophthalmology work in developing countries, which can often make the difference between a person being dependent and productive. Globally, the associations of disability with preventable social conditions – poverty and bad living conditions, tobacco, alcohol and unhealthy food, war, and unsafe work – show that much can be done to reduce the incidence of disabling health conditions.

UNDERSTANDING HEALTH NEEDS OF DISABLED PEOPLE

As well as their *primary impairment*, disabled people are at greater risk of *secondary impairments*, where one causes the other. For example, people with SCI are at increased risk of pressure sores and urinary tract infection. People with Down syndrome are more likely to experience congenital heart disease, impaired hearing and early onset dementia. People with schizophrenia are at higher risk of diabetes. Disabled people are also at higher risk of *co-morbidities*, where the cause is less direct. For example, nearly a third of people with a long-term physical condition have a mental health condition such as anxiety or depression. People with mental health conditions are more likely to experience obesity, smoking, heart disease, high blood pressure, respiratory disease, diabetes and stroke. Older people, for example those with dementia or stroke, are very likely to have more than one condition, which makes medical care more complicated. In general, disabled people have a *narrower margin of health*, for example they may be at increased risk of dying of influenza in an epidemic.

However, structural factors are as important as risks associated with having a disabling health condition. In particular, disabled people are also at higher risk of violence, as was discussed in earlier chapters. Disabled people also tend to be at higher risk of some unintentional injuries, such as falls or road traffic injury. Poor people have higher rates of long term illness, and disabled people are generally at risk of poverty, all of which means they are also more likely to experience other health risks associated with social disadvantage (e.g. poor housing and diet). Dangerous health behaviours may trigger health conditions associated with disability indirectly: e.g. drug or alcohol abuse may lead to disability as a result of road traffic injury.

Looking more closely at learning disabilities, evidence from the UK Learning Disability Observatory suggests:

- Less than 10 per cent of adults living in supported accommodation eat a balanced diet. Carers generally have a poor knowledge of public health recommendations on dietary intake.
- People with learning disabilities are much more likely to be underweight or obese than the general population
- 80 per cent of people with learning disabilities do not do enough physical activity (compared with 53–64 per cent of the general population).

Partly as a consequence, mortality rates among people with moderate to severe learning disabilities are three times higher than in the general population, with mortality being particularly high for young adults, women and people with Down syndrome.

The Health Improvement Project was a local intervention for people with learning disabilities funded by Norfolk and Waveney Public Health and run by Equal Lives, the disabled people's organisation for Norfolk. It was recognised by the Department of Health as a model of good practice in coproduction of services with people with learning disabilities. Key messages from the project included the following:

- People did not have support to cook for themselves, though they wanted to, and they did not know enough about eating healthily. Support workers also lacked knowledge of good diets, and time to cook better food.
- Gyms were inaccessible, and staff in sports facilities were not trained to include people with learning disabilities.
- There was a lack of awareness of the health checks which GP surgeries were meant to be offering people with learning disabilities.
- Smoking cessation programmes were not effective for people with learning disabilities: it was important to include an individual's circle of support, if they were going to successfully quit.

- Accessing sex education and sexual health information was a big priority for participants, many of whom had missed out on sex education at school.
- Mental health services were difficult to access, partly because there was often a conflation between the learning disability and the other mental health needs individuals might have.

The evidence from these two sources suggests that people with learning disabilities are at higher risk of ill-health, but much of this could be changed with some simple changes and interventions, such as more imaginative social support and more targeted health checks.

BARRIERS TO GENERAL HEALTHCARE

Disabled people experience a variety of barriers, when they try to access general healthcare – such as GPs or hospital services. These include physical barriers – such as the design of transport, buildings, or even examination couches, which may be hard to access for people with mobility impairments. Information can be a barrier – for example, for people who are blind or deaf or have cognitive limitations. Another barrier is the attitudes of healthcare workers. Research has shown that doctors are anxious about treating people with learning difficulties or mental health problems. There may not be time for a thorough consultation with someone who has complex problems or communication impairments. Less tangible are the systemic barriers, for example those arising from particular education policies or benefit regulations. All of these environmental factors can be reduced or mitigated.

At the global scale, the 2011 WHO *World Report on Disability* included analysis of the WHO World Health Survey which showed that globally people with disabilities were twice as likely to find healthcare provider skills or equipment inadequate to meet their needs; three times more likely to be denied care; and four times more likely to be treated badly, as compared with non-disabled respondents. The *World Report* also demonstrated how, particularly in low income settings, access to rehabilitation is often inadequate, both due to shortfalls in provision of trained doctors and therapists, and because of the lack of integration of rehabilitation services with primary health care.

In the UK, one might expect that there would be fewer barriers to healthcare, given that the NHS is free at the point of delivery, and that supply of trained personnel is better than in less developed countries. However, a range of problems contribute to the worse health outcomes which have been documented for disabled people. These include ignorant or negative attitudes among healthcare staff at all levels. Too many health providers fail to communicate adequately with the patient with disability themselves, for example seeking consent for procedures from the carer or relative rather than the person themselves.

For example, people with visual impairment may be reluctant to admit to their problems reading information, or may miss out on information. They may not be able to sign in via the screen at the doctor's surgery. Their independence and privacy may be undermined if they have to ask friends or relatives to read communications to them. At worst, they may make errors taking medications if they misread labels. A person with hearing loss may have difficulty making an appointment or may mishear their diagnosis. Deaf and hard of hearing people have told me about the Audiology clinic, where there is a verbal request for the next patient – who, by definition, is unlikely to hear his or her name being called.

Diagnostic overshadowing refers to the phenomenon where the primary condition becomes the focus of a consultation, rather than the general health problems a disabled individual may also be experiencing. Sometimes, people with learning disabilities find that symptoms of physical ill health are mistakenly attributed to either a mental health or behavioural problem. Again, lower uptake of health promotion and screening has been documented for disabled people, particularly for people with learning disabilities: for example, vision or hearing assessments, dental care, cervical smears, breast self-examination or mammography. People with learning disabilities who develop cancer are less likely to be informed of their diagnosis and prognosis, less likely to be given pain relief and less likely to receive palliative care.

Overcoming barriers to healthcare requires a number of actions:

1   Barrier removal – this means making healthcare premises and facilities accessible to wheelchair users. It also means meeting the communication needs of people who are visually impaired or have hearing loss, or who use sign language or who have learning disabilities. For example, better contrast or larger type makes it easier to read labels, or letters can be sent as digital or audio files rather than on paper.

2   'Reasonable adjustment' – a term which describes how changes can facilitate participation. This would include communicating in accessible formats with people with visual or hearing loss, for example via sign language interpreters. It might also mean giving longer time for consultations.

3   Training of healthcare workers – this can both challenge negative attitudes and assumptions, and also ensure understanding of the specific and general needs of disabled people.

4   Targeted interventions may be needed, such as specific clinic sessions for people with learning disabilities.

Overall, enhancing health literacy of disabled people and their family members can improve self-management and promote healthy life styles. Disabled people are often experts in their own condition, having lived with it for years, or even a lifetime. Therefore, partnership working between patient and professional has to be the way forward, rather than traditional doctor/patient approaches. In a time and cash constrained health system, it may be difficult to develop these understandings – not least because the patient may see a different doctor every time they make a consultation.

REHABILITATION PROVISION

Healthcare can be considered to entail four phases: prevention, cure, rehabilitation and maintenance. Rehabilitation is often neglected, despite playing a vital role in many cases where health conditions cannot be cured. In healthcare, rehabilitation is low status and low priority. In disability research, rehabilitation is over-looked, despite its vital role, for example in the lives of children with cerebral palsy, adults who experience spinal cord injury or head injury or stroke, or people of any age who become blind or deaf. Rehabilitation does not cure impairments, but it can prevent loss of function, slow the rate of loss of function, improve function, compensate for lost function, or maintain current function. Habilitation is a term which is often used in connection with rehabilitation services for children, for example those born with cerebral palsy, who may require physiotherapy or assistive devices in order to maximise their function.

Rehabilitation services and rehabilitation knowledge have historically been boosted in the aftermath of conflict, such as the First World War, the Second World War and the Vietnam War. Survivors of serious injury often had considerable residual disability, and their function was often greatly improved by targeted intensive rehabilitation programmes, including provision of wheelchairs, prosthetics and orthotics. The development of the disabled people's movements, and of rehabilitation sciences, often go hand in hand. For example, average life expectancy of people with spinal cord injury was around one or two years in the first half of the twentieth century. Building on the pioneering work of Donald Munro in 1930s America and Ludwig Guttmann in post-war Britain, life expectancy for people with paraplegia has now risen to approximately 90 per cent of that of non-disabled people. Most of the gains have been in reducing mortality from urinary tract infections and pressure sores, through better equipment and nursing care. With greater survival has come more participation – in Paralympic sports, but also in disability activism. More recently, there has been a revival of interest in military medicine (and with it, rehabilitation techniques) as a result of the twenty-first century wars in Iraq and Afghanistan.

Rehabilitation begins with thorough assessment of the disabled person's functioning. This allows clinicians to identify what can be done to restore or compensate for functioning loss, including what equipment or adaptations to the home or car or workplace might be empowering for the individual. This is the basis for the care plan which is agreed between the disabled person and the clinician. It is very important for the disabled person to become partners in their own rehabilitation, and education of the patient to self-manage is an important aspect of the rehabilitation plan. For example, an individual will have to do the physiotherapy exercises at home, as well as in the outpatient clinic. Third, the service will deliver the care plan. Rehabilitation operates via teams. In the NHS, the lead clinician is usually the specialist rehabilitation consultant. But they work closely with other doctors (orthopaedic surgeons, neurologists, etc.), as well as with therapists (physiotherapy, occupational therapy, speech and language therapy, psychology) and experts in assistive technology, such as wheelchairs, hearing aids, and assisted communication.

Assistive devices are very important in enabling disabled people to maximise their functioning. Moreover, advances in wheelchair technology have played a vital role in achieving independence, and even in the development of the disabled people's movement. The Everest and Jennings folding wheelchair, first devised in 1933, was a turning point. But up until the late 1960s, wheelchairs were big, heavy and clumsy. In 1979, the Quickie model of ultralightweight chairs transformed people's options – not only was it easier to use, it was also more stylish, coming in different colour options. These lightweight chairs also made modern Paralympic sports a possibility. Meanwhile, a new power chair was devised by George Klein in post-war Canada, in discussion with disabled veterans. As it became refined into a lightweight, fast machine, it has been similarly revolutionary for disabled people who lack the strength to push. In the developing world, since 1991 the international development NGO Motivation have pioneered the design and construction of cheap wheelchairs for rough terrain, reaching 80,000 people in more than 60 countries. Meanwhile WHO has offered guidelines for wheelchair provision in low income settings and associated training courses.

People can receive rehabilitation in different settings – acute in-patient hospitals, spinal cord injury or neuro-rehabilitation centres, outpatient clinics and in the community. People can receive rehabilitation immediately after an injury, or they might receive interventions at any point during the course of a long term condition such as MS or arthritis. Rehabilitation is not a one-off process. Today, in the NHS, there is a three-tier system: specialist settings in general hospitals; community teams, including specialised community MS teams or stroke early discharge teams; and then specialist spinal cord injury or head injury centres. For example, there are around 10 specialist spinal injury units in the UK, which cater for many of the thousand new cases each year, as well as looking after previous patients who return for further rehabilitation or care. Although rare, the physical, psychological, social and financial consequences of both of these types of disability are profound, which is why there are specialist services to ensure high standards of care for these patients. In all of these settings, a multi-disciplinary approach is taken, with physiotherapy, occupational therapy, speech and language therapy, psychology, social work and other input.

Globally, access to rehabilitation services is often very limited. Many sub-Saharan countries, for example, may only have one or two occupational therapists or speech and language therapists for the whole country. Worldwide, less than 15 per cent of people who need wheelchairs have an appropriate device. Without rehabilitation, people who are born or become disabled cannot participate in school or in livelihood activities, remaining dependent: death-rates from pressure sores and urinary tract infections are very high, for example for people with spinal cord injury. Community-based rehabilitation (CBR) is an approach which seeks to help disabled people living far from hospitals, harnessing the family and community to help the individual – not just with basic rehabilitation but also to access education, social and livelihood opportunities.

LEARNING DISABILITIES PROVISION

Services for children or adults with learning disabilities should be person-centred, and based on normalisation or equality principles. Normalisation means leading a life as close to that of non-disabled people as possible, with the same rights and entitlements. The philosophy of normalisation was pioneered in the Nordic countries, and then adopted by the Canadian, Wolf Wolfensberger, who developed it into his theory of Social Role Valorisation: it has underpinned much progressive practice in this field, but some people would prefer to follow the more recent development of human rights principles. Social services need to identify people with learning disabilities, but then the appropriate response requires multi-agency working and collaboration. Informal carers may need support, as well as the individual themselves, but the focus should be the person with learning disability.

My first job was working in a residential hospital for people with learning difficulties. Thirty years later, that hospital, like most others, has closed down, and the former residents are living in the community. In 2009, there were over 140,000 adults with learning difficulties in England. Thirty-seven per cent lived with family or friends; 18 per cent in care homes; 17 per cent in group homes; and 18 per cent were tenants or owner occupiers. Three per cent lived in adult placement situations such as the Shared Lives scheme, where an unrelated adult with learning difficulties lives with non-disabled people, who are paid an allowance. The rest lived in sheltered housing, nursing homes and hospitals.

In the last twenty years, there has been substantial progress in the policy response to people with learning disabilities, starting with the 2001 white paper *Valuing People*, which sets out the principles of equality of citizenship, advocacy and person-centred care for this much neglected group in the population. But despite these fine words, awareness grew over following years about failures in care for people with learning difficulties. For example, the Healthcare Commission (now superseded by the Care Quality Commission) investigated concerns about poor standards of care and abuse of people with learning disability in the Cornwall Partnership NHS Trust in 2006. It found poor practice, an unacceptable care environment and physical abuse of people with learning disabilities.

In 2007, the learning disabilities charity MENCAP publicised six case studies of avoidable death, and highlighted institutional discrimination against people with learning disabilities in the NHS. This led to Healthcare for All, an independent inquiry into access to health care, which led to recommendation to ensure that the NHS did not breach its duties under the Equality Act but instead provided 'reasonable adjustments' to ensure equal access to health services for people with learning disabilities. This included providing easy read communication and providing liaison nursing staff in hospitals, together with better processes to identify people with learning disabilities (although this itself is complex). NHS Trusts also had to report annually on progress. In 2009, the white paper *Valuing People Now* included new service priorities, building on these inquiries. Today, Learning Disability Partnership Boards are the structures which coordinate delivery of services.

Since this work, there have been several developments. Between 2010 and 2013, the Confidential Inquiry into the Premature Deaths of People with Learning Disabilities (CIPOLD; www.bristol.ac.uk/cipold) reviewed the deaths of 247 people:

- Nearly a quarter of these people with learning difficulties were younger than 50 years when they died, and the median age at death was 64 years.
- Median age at death of the men with learning difficulties was 65 years, 13 years younger than the median age at death for men in the general population of England and Wales.
- The median age at death of the women with learning difficulties was 63 years, 20 years younger than the median age at death for women in the general population.
- Avoidable deaths from causes amenable to change by good quality health care were more common in people with learning difficulties (37 per cent) than in the general population (13 per cent).

In 2011, the TV programme *Panorama* aired an investigation of Winterbourne View, a private hospital for people with learning difficulties, where patients were neglected and even assaulted and punished for their challenging behaviour. Complaints had previously been made to the Care Quality Commission, without effect. An enquiry followed, which led to Winterbourne View and several other facilities being closed down by CQC, and further investigations of many other institutions. Eleven workers from Winterbourne View pleaded guilty to charges of neglect and six were jailed. In addition, the head of the CQC resigned.

Another scandal was the 2013 death of 18-year-old Connor Sparrowhawk, who was living at Slade House, an NHS short-term assessment and treatment unit run by Southern Health. Connor was epileptic and autistic, but had been left unsupervised to have a bath: he drowned, after having a seizure. It was found that serious failings and neglect had contributed to his death. An audit of Southern Health found that 700 other deaths of people with learning disabilities or mental health problems from 2011 to 2015 had not been properly investigated. Seven years earlier, another patient had drowned in the same bath. Two years before this first death, a recommendation was made to remove the bath, but was never implemented. Connor Sparrowhawk's mother and friends led a high-profile campaign against Southern Health, and to highlight poor treatment of young people with learning difficulties in the health and care system.

In most English regions, social services are the lead agency for multi-disciplinary community teams which bring together learning disability nurses, social workers, therapists and other professionals to provide home visits to support people with learning disabilities and their families. This enables provision of advice, discussion of respite care, help with behaviour change, as well as coordinating other services and ensuring good communication and cooperation between agencies. Supported living arrangements to enable people to live in their own home, or with a peer or a small group, are developing, increasingly with the help of direct payments (individual budgets). However, some people still go into residential care, for example homes run by Mencap or other charities.

MENTAL HEALTH PROVISION

Not until effective drugs were discovered in the post-war period would mental health conditions like bipolar disorder and schizophrenia become manageable. Despite unwanted side-effects, successful drug treatments enabled many people with serious mental illness to come out of mental hospitals and live successfully in the community. Yet over this same period, the user movement of people with mental health conditions has grown in opposition to psychiatry, objecting both to forced treatment, and to drugs which leave many users lethargic and overweight. Challenging stigma, so that there is more understanding and acceptance of people affected by mental illness, will reduce exclusion, isolation and unemployment, and thus make it easier for people to live with these mental health conditions, to survive them, and to recover.

Towards the end of the twentieth century, cognitive and behavioural therapies were merged into cognitive behavioural therapy (CBT). In the early twenty-first century, these forms of psychological treatment have become widespread, based on the accumulating evidence of their effectiveness, particularly for common mental health problems such as anxiety, depression, eating disorders or obsessive compulsive disorder. For example, in the NHS, the Increasing Access to Psychological Therapies (IAPT) programme from 2008 has trained many psychological therapists to deliver courses of CBT. While short-term effects of CBT can be very good, these benefits wear off and the treatment needs to be repeated. There has also been some evidence that CBT has declined in its effectiveness over the years since it was first introduced, perhaps because practitioners are now less well trained, or because patients have lost faith in it.

Since the 1990s, the principle of service user involvement and expert patients has become more and more important in Britain's NHS. It can be argued that the development of service user initiatives has been influenced by prevailing political and social climates and that the promotion of user involvement in the industrialised world has coincided with the crisis in the funding of healthcare. In 2011 the World Psychiatric Association (WPA) stated a key goal for best practice when working with service users and carers is to promote meaningful involvement of users in the planning and implementation of services and the development of person-centred care.

A wide range of service user led activities exists throughout the world ranging from patient mutual support groups to projects staffed and managed by users. The recovery movement is not focused on curing symptoms, but on regaining hope, and finding ways to live positively. For example, Recovery colleges have been emphasised by service users as a good tool in recovery. They enable individuals to focus on their strengths rather than their problems, learn about themselves, their illness, and develop skills and tools needed for recovery. This approach was pioneered in Boston, USA, and is now present in services in Italy, Ireland and England. Another recovery movement concept is the principle of peer support, which was developed in the survivor movement, where individuals with lived experience of mental illness supported others in recovery. Now, many NHS mental health trusts employ service users as peer support workers, and the emerging evidence of their effectiveness is very good. People who sometimes have episodes of psychosis have used advance directives to create a joint crisis plan with healthcare professionals, which means that even when they are unwell or lack capacity, they can have confidence that their experiences and wishes regarding treatment will be respected.

For many people, mental illness is a chronic, long-term condition – much like other disabling impairments. Various approaches emphasise living well with mental illness, based on self-help and collaborative working:

- The Illness management and recovery (IMR) approach implements five core strategies; psycho-education, cognitive behavioural approaches, relapse prevention, coping and social skills training and is based on 5–10 months of individual or group training. The focus of IMR weekly sessions delivered by professionals is on self-directed problem defining and solving and the pursuit of personally meaningful goals.
- Wellness recovery action planning (WRAP) is used widely in the USA. A service user who is in recovery leads eight to twelve weekly sessions aimed at creating individual plans for recovery. Trials have found this leads to significant reductions in psychiatric symptoms and improvements in individual's hopefulness and quality of life.
- Particularly in German-speaking countries, mental health trialogues, otherwise known as psychosis seminars, are a community forum by which service users, friends, family, carers and mental health workers join in an open dialogue on various topics concerned with the challenges on being a service user.

While these service-user-centred activities emphasising community living and recovery are very important signs of progress in mental health services, it should also be emphasised that emergency care is also needed, when people become unwell. In the UK, the NHS funds physical care much better than it does mental illness care, despite the huge need for professional and evidence-based mental health care.

CONCLUSION

A human rights approach to disability does not negate the importance of health interventions including prevention, cure, rehabilitation and maintenance. However, disabled people will always be part of the population, and the necessary responses will be as much about barrier removal and equalisation as medical treatment. A just society is one which both removes barriers to the participation of disabled people, and which also meets the additional needs of those who cannot flourish in the mainstream. Health services and health professionals have an important role in improving the lives of disabled people. They should help fulfil the human rights of people with disabilities and provide reasonable adaptations to ensure that needs are met and dignity is respected.

Public health begins with identifying the number of people in the population who have health conditions associated with disability, but it should also include identifying disabling barriers. Assessing need at both individual and population level is a key prerequisite to the provision of appropriate services and requires attention to research and data collection. Services for disabled people will be most effective when they are based on good needs assessment and when they are founded on teamwork – both at the organisational (health, social services, voluntary sector) and at the individual level (doctors, nurses, therapists, social workers, family members). Above all, partnership between professionals and service users is required, both for the individual, but also at the policy level, where disabled people should be consulted on all matters which concern them, following the disability rights principle of 'nothing about us without us'.

FURTHER READING

Helen Atherton and Debbie Crickmore, editors. 2011. *Learning Disabilities: towards inclusion*. London: Churchill Livingstone Elsevier.

Public Health England. 2014. *People with Learning Disabilities in England 2013*. London: Public Health England.

Liz Sayce. 2016. *From Psychiatric Patient to Citizen Revisited: overcoming discrimination and social exclusion*. Basingstoke: Palgrave Macmillan.

World Health Organization. 2011. *World Report on Disability*. Geneva: World Health Organization.

World Health Organization. 2014. *International Perspectives on Spinal Cord Injury*. Geneva: World Health Organization.

EDUCATION FOR ALL

Education is critical to everyone, but particularly to disabled children. It is critical because having qualifications can make the difference to being included or excluded in employment and society. It is critical because disabled children may have special educational needs, which makes teaching and learning more complicated. It is critical because self-esteem and social capital are strongly influenced by educational experiences. Yet of all areas of disability policy, education is one of the most contested. Even the definitions in play reflect these debates:

- Segregated education is when children with disabilities are educated at special schools or home-schooled.
- Inclusive education means the child with special educational needs spending most of their day with non-disabled children in a mainstream school.
- Integrated education is when children attend special classes or units in mainstream schools.

Disability activists, many of whom received poor-quality education at segregated schools thirty or more years ago, always argue strongly for the pedagogical and social benefits of inclusion. Meanwhile, some parents of disabled children argue that their child's particular needs will never be met in a mainstream class-room, and that he requires targeted support within a small class, in order to maximise his potential. Other parents conversely argue that their child needs to grow up alongside non-disabled children in the mainstream. Lawyers support parents to achieve each of these contradictory outcomes by contesting schooling decisions at education tribunals.

Meanwhile, in low- and middle-income countries, many disabled children are not in school at all, missing out on the education which might mean the difference between a life of dependency and a life of productivity and independence. Education of disabled children is seen as a low priority in development, or as a problem too complicated to solve.

UNESCO's policy guidelines for inclusion state that the following are required to achieve inclusion:

- a recognition of the right of children with disabilities to education and its provision in non-discriminatory ways;
- a common vision of education which covers all children of the appropriate age range; and
- a conviction that schools have a responsibility to meet the diversity of needs of all learners, recognising that all children can learn.

In this chapter, I will trace the history of special education, discuss the debate between mainstream and segregated schooling, and then discuss provision in developed and developing countries. Along the way, I will try to say something about early intervention and about higher education, because it is wrong only to focus on schools, when disabled people, like everyone else, receive education before and after the compulsory years.

THE BEGINNINGS OF SPECIAL EDUCATION

Historically, disabled children, particularly those who were blind or deaf or had learning difficulties, were thought to be ineducable. With the Enlightenment, these views began to change. The first British school for deaf people was established in Edinburgh in 1760. Meanwhile, Abbe Charles Michel de l'Epee created the first institute for deaf education in 1784, using sign language, and Louis Braille devised his alphabet of raised bumps (1829). This opened up possibilities for the formal education of deaf and blind people. In nineteenth century France, Jean Marc Gaspard Itard tried to teach Victor, a 'wild boy', how to communicate and become more socialised. Although he had mixed success, one of his followers, Edouard Seguin later emigrated from France to the United States, where he developed guidelines for educating children with special needs.

At the turn of the century, other educational pioneers such as Maria Montessori and Ovide Decroly developed child-centred environments and approaches which facilitated independent learning and exploration by children. In the early twentieth century, as compulsory education for all was adopted in industrialised countries, separate classes for deaf, blind and learning disabled children began to be provided. After the Second World War, all developed countries organised systems of education for disabled people, parallel to the mainstream but separate from it. Special schools were also opened in developing countries, often by religious or other charitable initiatives. Many of these special schools, in developed and developing countries, were residential, taking children away from their families.

EARLY CHILDHOOD INTERVENTION AND PRE-SCHOOL

It is necessary to say something about early interventions before the years of compulsory education, the importance of which is increasingly recognised. Often, disabled children are disadvantaged even before they begin at school. Early childhood development interventions focus on mothers and children, considering the importance of the first 1,000 days of life for healthy neurological, social and emotional development. *The Lancet* has concluded that 43 per cent of children under 5 in low- and middle-income countries are at risk of not attaining their potential due to extreme poverty and stunting. Good diet, nurturing care and other environmental factors can make a huge difference to children in developing countries: absence of this care can result in stunting, deficits in language and cognition and problems in behaviour.

Early childhood intervention can also help reduce inequalities between high- and low-income families. A higher proportion of disabled children end up abandoned in orphanages or having poor quality care, with negative impacts on intellectual development and later achievement. Early childhood intervention programmes can make a difference to all children, but particularly to children who are deaf or who have autistic spectrum or other developmental conditions. China is one example of a county which has prioritised early childhood intervention for disabled children; 47 low- or middle-income countries provide early interventions to address developmental delays and conditions like autism and ADHD. Home visits by community health workers can improve parenting skills and promote health and nutrition, as well as reducing the risk of child neglect and other maltreatment. Since 2015, the Sustainable Development Goals have included children having access to high-quality pre-primary education, and this is particularly important for children with disabilities.

INCLUSIVE EDUCATION

In Britain, the philosopher and former head teacher Mary Warnock chaired a committee which brought out an influential report on special education in 1978. These recommendations formed the basis of the 1981 Education Act which was a landmark in inclusive education. While the Warnock Committee believed that 20 per cent of children might have some form of special educational need, they envisaged 2 per cent being eligible for a formal statement of special educational need, meaning that the child would receive additional specialist support. Local Education Authorities were given responsibility for the state-menting process and for ensuring children got the required support, either in the special school or mainstream sector. If parents were unhappy about this provision they could appeal, ultimately to the Secretary of State. Later legislation introduced Special Educational Needs and Disability Tribunals who would hear these cases – either when parents wanted a special school place or mainstream school place for their child, or wanted particular provision made. Legislation also strengthened the presumption that children would be educated in the mainstream.

Shifts in Britain echoed those in other parts of the world. In the United States, the landmark Education for All Handicapped Children Act was passed in 1975 to prohibit discrimination against disabled children and promote access to education. It was later modified to become the Individuals with Disabilities Education Act (IDEA), requiring special educational provision in the least restrictive environment for children from age 3 to 18 or 21. The equivalent of the UK statement of special educational needs is the Individual Education Plan (IEP). Evidence has shown that African Americans are disproportionately represented in the special education system, being three to four times more likely to be labelled as having learning difficulties in some US states, and to be more likely to be segregated from non-disabled children. This points to failings in the educational system as a whole.

In June 1994, UNESCO's World Conference on Special Needs Education adopted the Salamanca Statement and Framework for Action, part of which reads:

1 Every child has a fundamental right to education.
2 Every child has unique characteristics, interests, abilities and learning needs.
3 Education systems should be designed and educational programmes implemented to meet these diversities among children.
4 Students with special needs must have access to regular schools with adapted education.
5 Regular schools with an inclusive orientation are the most effective means of combating and preventing discriminative attitudes and building up an inclusive society.

ARGUMENTS ABOUT SCHOOL PLACEMENT

The main argument for educating all children together is one of equality. All children have the same rights, and the same basic needs to be supported, educated and to be with other children. It is important for all children to learn about difference, and to understand that although people are different, they are equally valuable. It can be very beneficial for non-disabled children to grow up with disabled children and understand diversity. Systems where black and white children are educated separately, or children from high socio-economic groups are educated separated, are divisive. Often, unequal resources get directed towards different groups. Often, one group is stigmatised, just as children who go to special schools are usually stigmatised, and grow up feeling more different. Even the 'favoured' group ends up worse off, because they are denied the chance to learn about difference and to develop more inclusive and accepting attitudes.

Where disabled children go to special schools, this often means travelling a great distance across town to the specialist provision – in rural areas, this may be even further. This may be difficult in itself – as well as exposing children to additional risk of abuse – and the corollary is that the child is less likely to know other children in their neighbourhood, because they all attend different schools. They may have fewer friends outside school.

This problem is even worse when the child is educated in a residential special school. They may be separated from their family for long periods of time from an early age. For example, in Africa I met many blind or deaf people who had gone to special school a long way away from their homes, and only been able to return to their families once or twice per year. The cost of obtaining an education was being emotionally isolated from parents and siblings.

Conversely, inclusive schools have to find new ways of teaching and learning and even moving around the school, that do not leave anyone behind. For example, some mainstream schools have realised that when everyone has the same break time, this leads to hundreds of children rushing along corridors and crowding in playgrounds. If children have different break times, there are fewer moving or playing at any one time, and this is beneficial for children with special needs who might otherwise be overwhelmed.

Another example is mixed age group classes. It is rare in human society for people of the same age to be clustered together. When grouped by age, the more able and less able stand out by contrast to their peers. People have different abilities and learn at a different pace. In a mixed age group class, this is recognised and supported. It is less noticeable that one 12-year-old is reading better than another 12-year-old, when the latter might be with 11-year-olds, and the former might be with 13-year-olds.

Segregation, it is argued, breeds segregation. While there may be a rationale for a very small number of children to receive targeted support, the existence of alternative provision becomes a rationale for segregating far more children where there is no practical or pedagogical need to do so. For example, not only children with learning difficulties, but also children with physical or sensory impairments might end up being segregated. Within the special system, there is further segregation. Diagnosis by an educational psychologist becomes critical. Different diagnostic groups get separated out for more specialist provision.

The majority of children can be educated with no adaptations. Where children do need special provision, this can be met within mainstream schools, in various ways. For example, a mainstream school might have a specific unit for children with special educational needs. A specialist mainstream school might offer bilingual teaching, so that deaf children can benefit from instruction in sign language.

Segregated schools are costly. Particularly in a developing country, it is not realistic to create enough special schools in all districts for all children who have special educational needs. Most children will either attend their local school, or be kept at home. Therefore, it is more practical to remove barriers and train teachers so they can include disabled children from the neighbourhood in the mainstream school.

However, a key argument for separate special education is that children with intellectual or emotional difficulties need provision which is targeted towards their specific needs for learning. Children who use sign language need sign language medium education. Children who are blind need materials and teaching approaches which are not based on visual methods. Specialist teachers with particular skills are available in special schools, as well as therapists and other professionals to help with speech, mobility and other needs, and the necessary equipment.

Another argument is about class size and school environment. Because children have additional needs, it is hard for these to be met within big mainstream classes. It would be better if they were taught in smaller groups, where they could get specialist attention.

The advantages of segregated education are that schools can be smaller in size than regular classes, with a higher adult-to-child ratio. The environment can be made accessible for all. Many children with autism and other behavioural conditions find large, noisy classes – or school playgrounds or corridors – to be over-stimulating and alarming, which tends to bring out their own more extreme behaviours. There may be a higher risk of bullying in a mainstream school.

Efficiencies result from children with the same impairment being brought together. For example, Deaf children can learn sign language and communicate with each other. It is plainly more cost effective to have all sign language using children in one school than to have to fund sign language interpreters to accompany every deaf child at his/her mainstream school. But it may also be more efficient to have tuition for blind pupils in the same place. If children are likely to need rehabilitation therapies, assistive devices or other interventions, such as a hydrotherapy pool, a special school can ensure that these are available during the school day to all children who need these services, whereas it may be more difficult to arrange sessions for children in mainstream schools.

Finally, if children with special educational needs are educated separately, there is no risk that the progress of non-disabled learners will be delayed or disrupted. Parents sometimes feel that disabled children in a class will take attention away from the non-disabled children. Children with emotional and behavioural difficulties may bully other children or make it more difficult for them to learn.

In practice, there are many compromises between entirely segregated education and entirely inclusive education. Children can attend special units or special classrooms within mainstream schools. They may spend part of their time with non-disabled children and part of the time in specialist classes. For example, there may be resource rooms for disabled children who are otherwise in mainstream classes.

It is important to realise that children are all different, and there may be different degrees of special educational need. Some children need remedial reading or arithmetic. Other children have dyslexia or a specific learning disability. Some children have mobility impairment, others have sight or hearing loss. Some children have intellectual impairment, to varying extents. Some children have emotional or behavioural difficulties. Provision for each of these needs may be different, and often can be met successfully in mainstream settings. The 2010 Special Educational Needs and Disability Review found that no one model – special school, inclusive school, special units in a mainstream school – worked better than any other. Good or bad provision could be found in any setting.

EDUCATION IN HIGH-INCOME COUNTRIES

In England, around a fifth of children have special educational needs. But the proportion of pupils with an Education Health and Care (EHC) plan, formerly known as a statement of special educational needs, is 2.8 per cent. The most common primary need among children is autistic spectrum disorder. Nearly 90 per cent of children with statements/EHC plans have learning difficulty or social, emotional and mental health difficulties, with the remainder having physical, hearing or visual impairments. Boys are nearly three times more likely to have a statement than girls. Pupils with special educational needs are more than twice as likely to be eligible for free school meals, and to have come from disadvantaged backgrounds.

In the UK, a number of reviews of special educational provision have come up with common themes for improvement:

- communication with parents;
- parental confidence in the system;
- early identification of needs;
- services that work around the family;
- joint work across professional boundaries;
- greater equity in access to additional provision; and
- the quality of training for staff, particularly for staff educating children and young people with the most complex needs.

The 2010 Special Educational Needs and Disability Review highlighted how improving the consistency and effectiveness of assessment of children was a key issue, particularly in avoiding different results in different areas of the country. Schools were too quick to label a child who was under-achieving as having special educational needs, when in fact they just required better teaching or higher expectations. Terminology in this field was found to be overly complex – 'special educational needs' versus 'disabled children and young people' versus 'children in need', for example, with different thresholds for assessing need in health, education and social care. The Review suggested that special education provision should be targeted on disabled children, with more focus on outcomes.

Outcomes for Deaf children in education remain problematic. In the most recent results, 41 per cent of Deaf children got five GCSEs (including Maths and English) at grades A* to C, compared with 57 per cent of other mainstream students. These results have not improved over the last six years, meaning that fewer Deaf children get the grades they need to access sixth form and higher education. Many Deaf adults have low literacy skills, with implications for employability.

Looking at education more widely, different countries have different educational policies, and hence different rates of segregated education. Nordic countries tend to have very inclusive systems, with most disabled children in the mainstream. Other countries still continue with largely segregated education. The European Agency for Special Needs and Inclusive Education (2013) data (www.european-agency.org) shows that out of 3,650,760 primary school pupils in England, 3,534,525 were educated in mainstream classes for at least 80 per cent of the time, leaving 112,330 in some form of segregated provision. This translates as about 3 per cent of English pupils in separate special schools. Conversely, in Sweden, out of a primary school population of 620,823, approximately 5,595 pupils have an official decision of special educational needs, of whom 4,856 are in separate special schools, translating as a rate of 0.7 per cent of Swedish pupils in separate schools. However, in the Flemish speaking part of Belgium, out of 432,402 children, 33,386 primary school pupils have a statement of special educational needs, of whom 18,481 are in separate schools. This translates as a segregation rate of over 4 per cent.

Disabled young people lack choices when it comes to post-school education. Particularly for low achievers, there are limited options available. Focus on the years of compulsory schooling obscures the importance of tertiary education. Most universities have made progress in removing barriers and improving access. Allowance is now made for students with specific learning disabilities, for example, extra time for exams. Although the UK Disabled Students' Allowance has been cut back in the austerity policies of recent years, it does meet some of the extra costs incurred by students with special needs, for example for specialist equipment, helpers – for example readers or sign language interpreters, travel and other costs.

At English universities in 2012–2013, there were:

- 16,600 students with mental health difficulties;
- 7,740 students with multiple impairments;
- 5,415 students with mobility difficulties;
- 4,085 students with hearing impairment;
- 3,845 students with a social or communication impairment;
- 2,260 students with visual impairment; and
- 80 students with autistic spectrum conditions.

However, these students were outnumbered by the 85,860 students with specific learning disabilities such as dyslexia. There were 1,287,865 students who had no known disability.

EDUCATION IN LOW-INCOME SETTINGS

How does this all play out in developing countries? The legacy of colonialism was a small number of charitable schools which helped a tiny percentage of disabled children learn, thrive and go on to prosper. Many leaders in the disabled people's movement attended such schools, particularly when they were deaf or blind. There they had tuition using braille, sign language or other modalities. They encountered disabled teachers who could act as role models. But as highlighted above, the cost of this residential special education was often being educated far away from their families. Moreover, the majority of disabled children in developing countries do not attend school at all: UNICEF suggests that a third of out-of-school children are disabled.

There are many barriers which explain the disparity. To start with, in rural areas, non-disabled children can walk for several miles to school, while many disabled children cannot do that. I remember meeting one man, Pius, in Zambia, who explained that he had been the only member of his family to finish school, despite his mobility impairment which meant he needed crutches to walk. It took him three hours to get to school each morning and each afternoon. Now he is chairman of his neighbourhood disability association, helping people with disabilities earn money through making furniture.

For those who make it to school, it is possible that they will find that their classroom is upstairs. Or they will find that there is no accessible toilet. I met a woman in Cairo who used a wheelchair; she could only attend school if she avoided using the toilet all day. When her classroom was upstairs, her classmates carried her in the wheelchair upstairs, at risk to their and her safety. Despite these barriers, she finished school, went to university, got a PhD, and she has now been elected to parliament.

For those who get to their classroom, and have a sight or hearing impairment, it is very likely that the teacher will lack the skills and equipment for them to be able to learn on an equal basis with others. They will probably be in a huge class of 80 children, making it very hard for them to get the attention they need. This numerical disadvantage also means that children with intellectual or behavioural impairments are likely to lose out. Teachers are often an obstacle to the inclusion of disabled children, because they feel that the presence of disabled children in the class will just make their job harder.

These factors make it very hard for disabled children to get the education they need in order to have any chance of making a living later on. Families often understand how important it is for the disabled child in particular to get qualifications. But the barriers, not least the cost of attending school, make it hard to succeed.

One argument for segregated provision is that special schools are barrier free, and have trained teachers. For those who can access them, they offer a chance of qualifications. For example, when I interviewed successful disabled people in Africa, a large number of them had attended segregated schools for blind or deaf children, often boarding schools a long way from their family. But the counter argument is that there will never be enough of these specialist schools to meet the need of all the disabled children. Therefore, pragmatically, the only chance is to ensure that mainstream schools are built to be barrier-free, to train teachers to be capable of teaching children with a range of needs, and to advocate for government policy to promote inclusion.

Turning to practicalities, working towards inclusion of disabled children means ensuring that those disabled children who are already attending school are not excluded from learning – for example, those blind or deaf children in large mainstream classes who need classroom assistants or educational materials in different formats. It means doing something about those children who are not attending, but could do so if schools were more flexible and welcoming. Extra resources are required for those children whose impairments mean they need additional support to learn.

At a systemic level, financial incentives – such as conditional cash transfers, where parents get payments if their children attend school – are a policy instrument which can promote educational inclusion. Transport subsidy might overcome some of the difficulties children have in accessing school. Schools can be provided with higher capitation fees for disabled pupils. Teacher training is key. There should be an element of special education as part of mainstream teacher training. Too few countries have effective policy and planning in place to ensure successful attainment by disabled children. Developing countries also need to collect data on disabled children, so they can make appropriate provision and assess achievement. Rather than special education being in the Ministry of Social Welfare, as often happens, it is very important for the Ministry of Education to oversee education of disabled children too.

At school level, having accessible premises, including bathrooms, means all children can participate. Having a trained focal point in each school means that other teachers can be assisted to include children with particular learning needs. Educational materials should be available in different formats for blind and deaf pupils. Classroom assistants can support children accessing education. Local disability groups can play a part in providing role models for disabled children and supporting parents.

There have been some great projects, often developed by international non-governmental organisations like Save the Children or Light for the World, which support inclusive schools, or work with national governments to provide inclusive education. For example, in 2001 Leonard Cheshire Disability began supporting five schools in Oriang, Kenya, to offer inclusive schooling to 500 disabled children out of several thousand pupils. This entailed ramps and toilets and levelling of ground; training for teachers; whole language approach to reading; community involvement. Yet there remain questions about sustainability at the end of this five-year project.

In Lao, Save the Children Norway worked with the government (1993–2009) to establish 539 inclusive schools, two or three in each district, which educated 3,000 disabled people alongside their peers. Government statistics (2007–2008) stated that the total number of school age children was 1,135,000 with total enrolled children with disabilities of 4,569, or about 4 per cent of the total. Given that on average around 5 per cent of children are disabled, these data appear impressive. However, again this was a time-limited project, and it is not clear whether all these gains were maintained in subsequent years.

These and other projects show what can be achieved, when the funding and the will is there. Education for disabled children is a problem which can be solved. Attitudinal change is needed, so that parents and teachers believe that disabled children have potential and can learn. Moreover, countries need to give inclusive education a higher priority, learn lessons from successful pilots, and take the steps to ensure that inclusive education is the routine, not the exception. This investment in disabled children will transform the prospects for disabled people. When I interviewed successful disabled people in four African countries, over and over again educational achievement was the common theme which accounted for them overcoming obstacles and becoming independent and productive adults.

CONCLUSION

Educating disabled children is among the best social investments, reducing welfare costs and future dependency, and improving the potential productivity of the disabled child. Currently, disabled children have lower educational attainment in both developed and developing countries. This means it is harder for disabled adults to escape poverty.

In high- and low-income countries, a key dimension of inclusive education is the attitudes of teachers and other professionals. These attitudes often depend on appropriate training and resources, and having had positive experiences of successful inclusion. Research shows that inclusion of disabled children has no adverse effects on non-disabled learners. What is good for children with special educational needs is good for all pupils, for example peer tutoring and cooperative learning. Again, assistive technology can be helpful to all children, but particularly to children with special educational needs.

Systems, not just individuals, are important. Accessible environments, for example, and the availability of early childhood intervention. Financing should provide incentives for inclusive provision. Monitoring and data collection are very important, to ensure that lessons are learned and good practice can be generalised. The best way to improve education for disabled children is to improve the education sector as a whole, with better training of teachers, smaller class sizes and better-resourced schools.

FURTHER READING

Ann Armstrong, Derrick Armstrong and Ilektra Spandagou. 2009. *Inclusive Education: International policy and practice*. London: Sage.

Maureen M. Black et al. 2017. Early childhood development coming of age: science through the lifecourse. *The Lancet* 389(10,064): 77–90.

Nidhi Singal, Roger Jeffery, Aanchal Jain and Neeru Sood. 2011. The enabling role of education in the lives of young people with disabilities in India: achieved and desired outcomes. *International Journal of Inclusive Education* 15(10): 1205–1218.

A MATTER OF LIFE AND DEATH

This chapter is about bioethics, a term which refers to the ethical and moral implications of biomedical practices and research. The field of bioethics brings together philosophers, lawyers, some social scientists and theologians, as well as clinicians and – not often enough – disabled people themselves. Here, I will focus on two key issues in bioethics: the beginning of life and the end of life. Unfortunately, this means overlooking other important bioethical questions, such as those about cures for illness and impairments, about limits to biotechnology, or about resource allocation.

Within bioethics, disability has tended to be seen in predominantly medical terms. Disability is often regarded simply as a deficit or difficulty of body or mind, under the care of doctors, and by association as a problem which can only be solved through medical intervention. As we have seen, there is a great fear of and ignorance about disability among non-disabled people, and bioethicists are not immune from this. Disability has predominantly negative associations: lack, pain, limitation, suffering, death. These ways of thinking affect how bioethical issues around disability are often conceptualised, at least within the secular liberal tradition.

The utilitarian and libertarian strands of bioethics generally receives the greatest attention in the media: think of writers like Peter Singer, Julian Savulescu, John Harris or Jeff McMahan, all of whom have written challenging, indeed provocative, interventions about disability. These moral philosophers seem to consider themselves more rational, more logical, more consistent, than others – meaning members of the public or even the medical profession. Often, this steers them towards vegetarianism, support for humanitarianism, and opposition to war and guns. But rather than being dominated by sentiment, religious doctrines about the 'sanctity of life' or other confused thinking, these thinkers also want us to rethink our approaches to some key bioethical questions.

For example, not only do they endorse prenatal screening and selective abortion, they have sometimes also argued that this should be permitted both up to birth, and in the neonatal period, if a fetus or newborn is 'severely impaired'. One notorious book was titled *Should the Baby Live?* They talk sometimes of the duty of 'procreative benevolence' – that parents should have the best children they can. None of these thinkers would seek to be proscriptive – they all support the principle of autonomy, which differentiates them from the eugenicists of the early twentieth century. But they would argue against restrictions on reproductive autonomy and urge prospective parents to take advantage of whatever information genetics and obstetrics can provide, and to act to have the 'best' children they can.

Disabled people who are active in research and activism generally stress other arguments. Following the social model approach to disability, impairments are better regarded in terms of difference, rather than deficit. Activists make the point that disability is strongly influenced by social factors: the type of society one lives in, the environmental barriers one encounters, the cultural representations and psychological attitudes one faces. Disabled people may face added difficulties from their health conditions, but these do not undermine their chance of leading a good life. The empirical evidence shows that disabled people generally enjoy a quality of life which is as good as, or sometimes better than, that of non-disabled people. Parents of children with Down syndrome, for example, stress the good lives they lead and joy they bring. Often, social factors, not the health condition, cause the greatest problems, and therefore disability rights advocates argue that attention should be directed to the alleviation of social factors, not the prevention or cure of health conditions. Disabled bioethicists such as Jackie Leach Scully or Joe Stramondo argue that disabled people often have not just a different attitude to disability, but also a different perspective on bioethical debates, because of their lived experience. It is important, not just for disabled people to explore ethical questions, but also for non-disabled people to understand more about the life of a disabled person.

BEGINNING OF LIFE

I do not approach the question of prenatal diagnosis with a firm sense that screening or selective abortion are morally wrong or socially undesirable, or that they risk returning us to a eugenic past, or even that they are potentially damaging to the human rights of people with disabilities. I support reproductive autonomy, as a principle. But when we explore the lived experience of prenatal diagnosis, it shows how screening and testing can be a mixed blessing, rather than simply beneficent.

Accounts in the media, and in popular science, whether presented by scientists themselves or by other commentators, often represent genetic testing, especially prenatal diagnosis, in terms of empowerment. Whereas in previous generations, people had no choice about reproduction, the claim is that now science has created technologies which provide prospective parents with information, which empowers them to make choices, thereby to promote the health of their families. Often, the emphasis in these accounts is on the hard science – the tests, the markers, the probabilities – rather than the human sciences – patient information, counselling, support – which are just as important if patients are to make informed choices, minimise harm and anxiety, and emerge from the process feeling resolved and empowered, not bruised and bewildered.

But despite this positive rhetoric and the expenditure of billions of dollars on the Human Genome Project, genetics has so far had limited impact on human health. Concrete outcomes – whether therapies or pharmaceuticals or other interventions – are slow in arriving. Knowledge, so confidently proclaimed at the point of the sequencing of the human genome, turns out to be less complete and more uncertain than previously imagined. The simple rules of Mendelian genetics are most relevant to rare single gene diseases (think of muscular dystrophy or cystic fibrosis) while common complex conditions (think of heart disease or dementia) which mainly occur late in life, turn out to be multifactorial, depending on many genes interacting with the environment, lifestyle and other factors. The details of gene expression and regulation, and the interaction of genes with genes, or genes with environment, appear to be ever more complex.

Despite the attention given to the NHS fetal anomaly screening programme, so far, few conditions can be diagnosed prenatally. The major application of testing is testing of biochemical markers and chromosomes for Down syndrome and other trisomies rather than any genetic analysis. Prenatal diagnosis via DNA is only offered when a family is at known genetic risk because parents are carriers of a recessive or X-linked condition, such as cystic fibrosis or muscular dystrophy. Diagnostic ultrasound, which can detect fetal structural anomalies, such as spina bifida or heart defects, is probably more relevant to fears of eugenics than any DNA based technology.

Pre-implantation genetic diagnosis (PGD), or embryo selection *in vitro*, is an extremely rare process, which (at least in the UK) is regulated closely by the Human Fertilisation and Embryology Authority (HFEA). Currently, PGD is only offered to couples who have had a prior child die of a diagnosable genetic disease. The numbers of people undergoing PGD have not radically increased in the years since the technique was invented in 1990.

These current limitations of genetic knowledge undermine both the more optimistic scenarios about health benefits arising from genomics, but also the more apocalyptic scenarios painted by critics of genetics. However, 'cell-free DNA' is a new development which may have far reaching implications. A simple maternal blood test can cast some light on the genetics of the fetus. At present, this non-invasive prenatal testing (NIPT) helps improve the risk calculation for women who are found to be at higher risk of Down syndrome or other trisomies after serum screening and ultrasound. Because NIPT is a much more accurate test, it can reduce the number of women who are referred for invasive testing, for example amniocentesis. In turn, this reduces the risk of miscarriage, which can be a very rare side-effect of invasive testing. However, NIPT is a screening test not a diagnostic test, so women who are found to be at higher risk still have to have the invasive test. NIPT can also be used for families at higher risk of inherited genetic conditions – muscular dystrophy or achondroplasia (restricted growth), and in these cases it can be diagnostic. Although at present, NIPT is only used for these eventualities, there may come a day when NIPT is combined with genome analysis to give accurate predictions of many different genetic conditions or traits, early in pregnancy.

The loudest currents in Anglo-American bioethics adopt rather shallow reasoning around prenatal diagnosis. Many ethical judgements rely on the famous 'four principles' outlined in the introductory bioethics textbook by Tom Beauchamp and James Childress, drawing on the traditions of Kantian deontology and Anglo-Saxon utilitarianism. These four principles – beneficence, non-maleficence, autonomy and justice – are meant to play an equal role in this normative toolbox. But in practice the value of autonomy predominates. In other words, decisions about prenatal diagnosis should be made by the prospective parents and choice should be upheld. But it is important to pay attention to the social context and the cultural climate in which 'choices' are made, because there are reasons to be sceptical about the possibilities of people deciding for themselves.

Religious or traditional thinkers would prefer to talk in terms of the sanctity of life or the moral value of the embryo. But secular thinkers reject these approaches, and appeal to the human desire for healthy and happy children. The majority of the population support abortion rights and a woman's right to choose. Is it not inconsistent to support the right of women to terminate pregnancy because they do not want to be pregnant, and then to oppose abortion on the basis of characteristics of the fetus? Again, most people would be in favour of measures to improve health and reduce impairment and illness – for example, taking folate in pregnancy to reduce the risk of spina bifida, or vaccinating an infant to reduce the risk of polio. Is it not inconsistent to support attempts to avoid existing people becoming impaired, but object to attempt to prevent the existence of impaired future people? Logic and consistency suggest that some of the arguments used by disability rights thinkers do not work.

Against those who would claim that disability is simply a different way of life, or that the main problems for disabled people are generated by environmental barriers or structural inequality, libertarian bioethicists such as Professor John Harris argue that disability is 'a harmed condition one has a logical preference not to be in'. Those disabled people who would insist otherwise are mistaken: their subjective feelings have got in the way of the objective fact that it is better not to have Down syndrome, spina bifida or visual impairment because these conditions either cause suffering, or limit opportunities.

I would suggest a more nuanced approach to evaluating the effects of prenatal diagnosis is required, because neither scientific triumphalism nor bioethical perfectionism attends to the emotions and feelings of key participants in the debate. The impact of testing and termination on women is complex. For some, testing offers reassurance, control and relief. To many, it makes the experience of pregnancy a more anxious time, whatever their decisions or choices around diagnosis. For a minority, it creates a situation where they have to choose whether to terminate a wanted pregnancy. And here the difference between general support for abortion rights and specific concern around selective termination becomes relevant: most social terminations, when a woman does not want to have a baby, occur in the first few months of pregnancy. In contrast, termination on grounds of fetal abnormality comes after 16 weeks in a wanted pregnancy: the woman wants to be a mother, but feels unable to become mother of this child. The emotional consequences of these two decisions will often be very different, as will the longer term feelings of guilt and pain for many women. For this reason, technologies which bring the diagnosis and decision-making earlier in pregnancy – such as non-invasive prenatal testing – become emotionally and morally important. Whether early or late in pregnancy, there remains a lack of research on the psychological sequelae of termination of wanted pregnancies.

The other stakeholders in the diagnosis debate are disabled people. There are many examples of criticism by disabled people and organisations of trends towards prenatal diagnosis. Sometimes, these challenges have been inflammatory and rhetorical, accusing proponents of genetic screening of being eugenicists or having parallels with the Nazis. Not all of the arguments have been consistent or sound. But rather than rejecting disability critiques as hysterical or ill-informed, it is preferable to understand the feelings of hurt and rejection which underlie these challenges.

As a result of the popularity of genetics, disabled people risk once more being defined as medical abnormalities and invalids, rather than as citizens, or victims of injustice. They see measures being implemented to prevent the birth of others with their conditions. They might think of whether their own parents would have taken advantage of such technologies. They might consider differential treatment of fetuses with and without disability to be discriminatory: in UK, termination is illegal after the 24th week of pregnancy, except in case of severe abnormality. No matter if these late terminations are very rare: the message has been sent that it is better to be dead than disabled.

What I am describing here has been labelled the 'expressivist objection', the idea that prenatal diagnosis 'expresses' a negative valuation of the lives of people with disabilities. The late Adrienne Asch, the disabled bioethicist who popularised this phrase, said that screening was an example of the literary device of 'synecdoche', taking a part for the whole. Rather than seeing the whole future person, genetic testing highlighted only the aspect of disease. Here, I want to draw attention not to the validity of the claim, but more to the actual feelings and reactions of disabled people. 'Expressivism' is not necessarily rational or logical, but it is important. Whether one views these hurt feelings as justified or mistaken, they exist and are another example of the damage done to human lives by the increased availability of prenatal diagnosis, and the wider discourse surrounding it. Disabled people are not necessarily criticising particular decisions, but often are expressing deep concern about the general 'direction of travel' of reproduction and pregnancy, with screening out disability increasingly considered as an issue of quality control.

There is also some evidence that attitudes to disability change, as a result of the advent of screening: Down syndrome, for example, becomes not a random accident or act of God, but something which could have been prevented. Families with Down syndrome children may be felt blameworthy. In some health and welfare regimes, this might be treated as 'elective disability', not entitled to coverage from private or social insurance. There might be less research and clinical expertise available, in future, to contribute to better lives for people with Down syndrome or other conditions, as they become rarer. Strangers in the street might look askance at the choices of someone who could have avoided this undesirable outcome, even when in fact this may have been impossible – for example, screening does not always work, there are 'false negatives' when the condition is not diagnosed in time.

I have never forgotten anthropologist Rayna Rapp's comment, 'This technology makes every woman into a bioethicist', referring to amniocentesis in her 1999 book, *Testing the Woman, Testing the Fetus*, an empirical account of decisions about prenatal diagnosis. She sums up how many (but not all) women and men deal with difficult decisions around testing and termination in pregnancy. Of course, there are those who will be business-like and unemotional about screening and diagnosis, welcoming the opportunity to be informed and take control. But I suspect that there are many others who worry about what to do, and agonise about whether it is morally or religiously justified to test or to terminate. They will ask themselves questions about whether it is right to use this power, about what makes life worth living, about what to do in the best interests of the potential baby, their other children, their marriage or their own life. They will worry about the act itself, and about the consequences of the act: would they regret it, either way?

This suggests and highlights how choice itself can be problematic. In the past, people did not have this level of power and control over their pregnancies, which was both bad and good. Now, people can take responsibility for something which previously was left to chance, God or karma. Potentially, the 700,000 UK pregnancies each year expose 1.4 million potential parents to screening anxiety and the burden of choice. In my discussions with couples, parents of disabled children often reflect that they are glad they did not have to make such a choice. They love and value their disabled child, and do not regret the outcome. In previous generations, once safe and reliable contraception was available, prospective parents could only control the number and timing of their children. Now they can increasingly influence the nature of their children, a move from quantity to quality control. Sometimes, ignorance is bliss.

Bioethical and biomedical versions of prenatal diagnosis also fail to account for the complexity and vulnerability of human embodiment. The drive for the 'perfect baby' will never eliminate disability, because frailty and impairment are a fact of life. While a small number of conditions can be detected, and potentially screened out, this leaves many other sources of variation and vulnerability. Genetics reveals that every genome carries within it at least one hundred mutations. Those who appear 'normal' may be predestined to disease, or have a higher risk of cancer, dementia or heart disease. Moreover, neonatologists are increasingly good at saving the lives of premature babies, up to half of whom will end up as disabled people.

Discourses on disability and diagnosis sometimes imply a polar dichotomy between the normal baby, for whom upbringing is plain sailing, soon to become independent, from the start a source of pride; and the baby with disability, destined to be a disappointment and a burden. Yet all children are, in some ways, a burden and also a joy. Even choosing the 'best fetus' cannot guarantee that your child will be free from impairment or illness. Approximately 1–2 per cent of births are affected by congenital disability while between 10–20 per cent of people are disabled: the majority of disability arises not from genetic causes but from lifestyle, disease and other environmental factors. Accidents are the highest cause of childhood mortality and morbidity.

Investment in the science and technology of diagnosis and screening has outstripped investment in the softer but equally important work of training, communication, counselling and support. This means that the rhetoric of choice conceals failures of provision which imperil ethical practice. For example, there is a lack of balanced information about the conditions for which testing is offered. Prospective parents are not necessarily told about life with a disability, and the possibilities for support and inclusion: instead, communication focuses on symptoms and limitations. Testimony from people with disabilities is rarely if ever included. At present, the NHS mainly presents information via a leaflet: in the age of websites and online video, this seems a major deficiency.

Despite an ethic of non-directiveness, sometimes doctors and other clinicians exert explicit or implicit pressure on their patients. This is especially the case in countries where the ethic of informed individual choice is less strong, and where there is a tradition of medical paternalism. Even where information and attitudes are better, there is often a conveyor belt impetus to pregnancy management, together with an unavoidable pressure of time, which makes it difficult for prospective parents to think through their choices and come to an informed decision. Each decision seems to pre-empt the one that comes next. The choice to have serum screening dictates the decision to have a follow-up diagnostic test if the pregnancy is found to be 'high risk' and the only action on receipt of a 'positive' test result is termination, an outcome which might not have been imagined at the beginning of that course of events.

In outlining these deficiencies, I am not calling for an end to choice or provision of information and services, but for better and more careful approaches to prenatal screening and testing. More and balanced information is badly needed, together with offers of counselling and support. Not all parents may wish to avail themselves of these options. The goal is for people to make decisions which feel right for them and which, as far as is possible, they do not regret later; no matter how much they continue to feel distress. It is as important to spend time and money not just on the science and technical issues of which markers and when to test on information, but also on sufficient information, counselling and support. If the ethic underlying screening is parental choice, then this must be a real choice, where people are supported to test, and not to test, to terminate, and not to terminate. Society must be willing to welcome disabled babies into the world. Otherwise it is not a genuine choice.

The discussion of screening in bioethics or popular science also obscures the failures of prenatal diagnosis: the false positives, the false negatives, the iatrogenic miscarriages which are an inevitable aspect of the process. In UK, almost all pregnancies are screened for raised risk of Down syndrome instead of, as was the case before, only the pregnancies of older women. Ninety-nine per cent of pregnancies which serum screening identifies as being at raised risk turn out to be unaffected (false positives). The diagnostic test which follows a positive screen is amniocentesis which, according to the Royal College of Obstetricians and Gynaecologists, carries an additional spontaneous termination risk of around 0.5–1 per cent. This means that for many women, their chance of being found to have a pregnancy affected by Down syndrome will be approximately the same as their chances of losing the pregnancy because of the diagnostic test. In addition, there are families who receive reassurance from screening or testing that their pregnancy is not affected, who then go on to have a baby with disability (false negatives). Research suggests that these false negatives can be harder to deal with than the unexpected birth of an affected child in the absence of screening.

Many prospective parents – up to one third – refuse the offer of prenatal diagnosis. Of those who accept the offer and then have a positive diagnosis of fetal anomaly after a diagnostic test such as amniocentesis, just over 90 per cent opt for termination. However, babies with Down syndrome continue to be born. The major factor underlying this is an increase in women having children later in life, because maternal age is a major risk factor for Down syndrome, just as advanced paternal age is implicated in certain genetic mutations. The conjunction of these trends explains the interesting fact that the birth-rate of children with Down syndrome has not fallen markedly, despite the heavy investment in diagnosis. What has been avoided has been the major increase in number of children with Down syndrome which might otherwise have resulted. Coupled with rising rates of infertility and consequent assisted reproduction techniques, this phenomenon highlights how changing social choices have necessitated increasing technologisation of conception and pregnancy. It also suggests that interventions should focus on supporting people with Down syndrome, not simply eliminating them.

So, where will it all end? The rapid pace of medical and scientific change causes alarm among some members of the public, and particularly among disabled people. While it is impossible to be certain about the near future, let alone what will occur in fifty years, there are some suggestions that could be made.

On the positive side, it is likely that it will be possible to test pregnancies earlier and more safely, for example with the use of NIPT at ten weeks of pregnancy, rather than waiting for ultra-sound and amniocentesis at 18–20 weeks. In other words, perhaps fewer late abortions and fewer miscarriages, with all the associated trauma and distress. With NIPT, the sensitivity and specificity of testing will continue to improve, reducing the numbers of both false positives and false negatives. And evidence from pilot research suggests that after NIPT and diagnosis of Down syndrome, more women choose to continue their pregnancy.

On the negative side, it is likely that more possibilities for testing and choosing will open up, as it is already beginning to happen with newborn screening and single nucleotide polymor-phisms (SNP) technology for late-onset diseases. If NIPT continues to improve, and is used in association with panel testing, or even whole genome sequencing, then potentially pregnancies could be tested for hundreds of conditions, not the few that are currently possible. These innovations will begin in the commercial sector, and then the NHS will come under pressure to adopt the same approach in order to ensure equality of provision.

Genome sequencing is becoming cheaper and faster, due to technologies such as parallel sequencing by synthesis and the use of nanowire or nanopore methods, often labelled 'next-generation sequencing'. This means that parents are more likely to know their carrier status in relation to recessive conditions before conception, and hence what potential risks their pregnancies might carry. It also means that it is quicker and easier to test fetal cells for more conditions, for example through non-invasive prenatal testing at ten weeks. Unrestricted testing would lead to prospective parents getting a huge amount of information that creates risk and uncertainty and does not give clear answers, for example with the many 'variations of unknown significance'. It could also lead to selection against many variants and in favour of embryos or fetuses which are 'disability free'. For this reason, I believe that there should be a moratorium on using whole genome sequencing for the foreseeable future.

If assisted conception techniques improve, it may be that more parents opt for pre-implantation diagnosis (PGD), which opens up many more possibilities for testing and selection, when it is combined with whole genome sequencing. For example, it seems very unlikely, within current context of ethics, law and clinical guidance, that selective termination would be performed for sex selection or to avoid late-onset conditions or to avoid fetuses which are carriers of recessive conditions, at least in western democratic societies. However, all of these possibilities are already happening in the case of pre-implantation genetic diagnosis, albeit in very few pregnancies. This technology is currently aimed at known carriers of fatal childhood diseases and some carriers of late-onset conditions such as Huntington's disease and heritable forms of breast and colon cancer. But its expansive potential is high, if used with whole genome sequencing. Currently, pre-implantation genetic diagnosis and assisted conception are unreliable and complex techniques, meaning that many couples have to decide between the risk of an affected baby (with normal conception) or no baby (with assisted conception).

With embryo selection or other advanced diagnostic approaches, the relationship of parent to child may change. Extra choices bring additional responsibilities. When I was part of a team researching how lay people felt about PGD, there was a strong sense that, while it was acceptable to use diagnosis to avoid disease, it was highly questionable as a method of choosing other characteristics of a child. People often talked in terms of children being 'a gift not a commodity'. Many mainstream bioethicists might say that, like the so-called 'yuck factor', this opposition arises from public unfamiliarity with these techniques and capabilities. Or maybe it captures something important about reproduction which our emphasis on choice and control is in danger of obscuring.

END OF LIFE

In thinking about assisted dying, my starting point is the values of the disability rights movement. One in seven of the population are disabled in some way, even though a tiny minority is actively involved in disability politics. The disability movement argues that disabled lives have value. Disabled people can contribute to society. Through their relationships with others and in many other ways they lead good lives that should be supported and celebrated. This is a radical claim. Rather than looking at achievements or qualifications or salaries or status, disabled people want to be regarded as people in their own right, as worthy of respect and dignity.

It is unfortunate that the politics of disability have not been more inspiring for the politics of old age. There has not yet been an equivalent older people's movement alongside the disabled people's movement, and many older people have been unpersuaded by disability rights thinking. Yet the refusal to be subject to medical domination, the determination to achieve choice and control, the demand for inclusion and respect, are all relevant to older people, with and without disability, and they could be influential in the debate on assisted dying. It's very encouraging to see that advocates are beginning to develop a disability-inspired human rights approach to dementia, for example.

It's not always easy for people with impairments or illnesses to recognise themselves as disabled people and feel pride and self-worth. Many children with disabilities are brought up to feel second-class, to feel dependent, and to be grateful for any help they can get. Many people who develop disability in adulthood – perhaps through sudden injury or acquired disease – take time to adapt and accommodate. The first reaction to traumatic or acquired disability is dismay. People often feel suicidal – I know I did, when I became spinal cord injured. It is hard to get used to not being able to do things that previously were taken for granted. Yet, as discussed in Chapter 3, the evidence shows that people do come to terms and return to their previous quality of life. This concept is known as 'hedonic adaptation', and is a very heartening example of how good human beings are at dealing with profound life changes.

Second, disabled people have argued for their human rights to be recognised, and demanded services and inclusion on the basis of these rights. The 2006 UN Convention on the Rights of Persons with Disabilities enshrines these rights. More than 170 states, including the United Kingdom, have ratified this Convention and are therefore bound to respect and promote these rights.

The Convention is predicated on the radical idea that people are disabled by society as much as by their bodies. That's why concepts such as equality and discrimination, access and attitudes are highlighted in the first few articles. It is often the barriers that are put in the way of disabled people which prevent them leading good lives or being included in education, employment, housing or leisure opportunities.

Central to these human rights is the principle of 'nothing about us without us', the principle that disabled people should be listened to and regarded as the experts on their own lives. Disabled people have argued strongly for choice and control over their own lives. Historically, disabled people have been spoken for by others. They have been passive recipients of care. Non-disabled people have often been motivated by pity. As a result, disabled people have lacked dignity and autonomy. That's why the principles of independent living have been so important. Even when severely impaired, people have been able to employ their own personal assistants to live independently in their own homes, participating in the community. These principles have now been eroded by 'welfare reform', and many disabled people fear being returned to the residential institutions from which they escaped in the 1970s and 1980s.

Third, disabled people also remember their history of eugenics and euthanasia. Not just in Nazi Germany, but in all of Scandinavia and many parts of the United States and Canada, disabled people were sterilised, particularly those labelled as 'feeble minded'. Under the Third Reich, this hatred of 'useless eaters' or 'lives unworthy of life' went as far as active euthanasia, with several hundred thousand children and adults with mental health conditions or learning difficulties being exterminated in gas chambers, by lethal injection, by machine gun or by neglect. So disabled people have experience of being treated in an evil way by society, with doctors as the agents of their discriminatory treatment.

These competing principles influence disabled people's attitudes to assisted dying in different ways. Some disabled people are adamantly opposed to any liberalisation of the law. They cite the history of eugenics and involuntary euthanasia, fearing that even a narrow and restrictive liberalisation will be the first step on a slippery slope. They highlight how the majority of the population have at best patronising, and at worst eugenic, attitudes to disability. They make the point that people newly disabled will share these negative valuations, and will feel that their own lives are not worth living. They fear that disabled people will feel pressurised by other family members to end their own lives, without exploring the possibilities of independent living, personal assistance and lives supported by assisted technology. After all, thousands of disabled people are living good lives, despite relying on machines to breathe, or assistants to bathe and feed them.

Yet other disabled people point to the disability rights movement value of choice and control. If we campaign for independent lives, should we not also campaign for autonomy at the end of life? Rather than having a difficult, lingering death, why not decide for oneself when enough is enough? If we believe that disabled people can decide for themselves, why can they not be permitted to decide about this most important question?

Central to a disability rights support for assisted dying is a differentiation between people living with disability, and people in end stage of terminal illness. It seems to me that it would be very wrong for any person who is disabled automatically to have the right to die. Death is not the answer to disability. When I hear of a young man who has become spinal cord injured travelling to Zurich to die in the Dignitas scheme, I feel very sad. Because the evidence is that disabled people can have a quality of life as good as non-disabled people, and sometimes even better. The data show that within a few years of sudden injury, quality of life returns to what it was before disability struck.

However, where someone is already dying, with a disease such as motor neurone disease or terminal cancer, it seems irrational to deny to them the right of a better death. The outcome is not changed: they would be dead within months anyway. They are not giving up on the possibilities of a long and fulfilled life, because they might have less than a year to live. Independent living is barely relevant, because no amount of accessibility or support services can compensate when one is struggling to breathe, or eat, or else enduring constant pain. The principle of equality is appropriate: if a healthy person wanted to end their life through suicide, they would be able to perform that act. But this terminally ill person, living at home or in hospitality in a state of complete debility, is highly unlikely to be able to end their own life. Hence the need for assistance.

The counter-argument from colleagues like (Baroness) Jane Campbell is that sometimes disabled people already have a terminal diagnosis: they are not expected to survive spinal muscular atrophy (SMA) or muscular dystrophy (MD) or multiple sclerosis (MS) in the long term. If they have a sudden crisis, perhaps pneumonia, they may be thought of as being in the end stage of their disease. 'Do not attempt resuscitation' (DNAR or DNR) may be placed on their hospital notes. So the two categories, of disabled people living independent lives, and terminally ill people experiencing a slow death, are sometimes hard to differentiate. Yet we come back to the principle of autonomy. Assisted dying should never be something that is imposed on someone. It should be something that is chosen by someone who knows that life is futile because they are inevitably going to die in weeks or days. This does not apply to people with SMA, MD or MS.

It seems very sensible that people are more likely to be having conversations about death with their loved ones. The Death Café movement is a good example of this. We should know what our partners, parents and siblings want to do at the end of life: whether they want to be organ donors or not; whether assisted dying is in line with their values, or not; what sort of treatment they would want to receive. Of course, people fear disability, almost as much as they fear dying. People may say they would rather be dead than endure dependency, but then when dependency happens, they discover that it's not the worst way to live, and that life can have value. That's why it's important to go on having those conversations, and to hear from the person directly affected about what's good and bad about their existence. That's why I also support the concept of 'Advance Directives', which allow someone to say what they wish to happen to them in future, if they are unable to decide for themselves.

Very few people will wish to avail themselves of assisted dying, based on the evidence from Oregon. In 2013, there were 31 assisted deaths per 10,000 deaths (a total of 105 people in Oregon). So after 15 years of the legislation, the number of people who took advantage of it represented 0.31 per cent of all deaths. But many, many, more will have been given extra courage in facing death by the knowledge that there is an easier way out, if they wish to take it.

I do not believe that this threatens disabled people, as long as safeguards are in place. The analysis of effects of the legislation in Oregon and The Netherlands is that vulnerable groups – such as disabled people, older people, women, poorer people, people with histories of psychiatric illness – are not unfairly impacted. From Oregon, we also know that the median age of people who chose assisted dying in 2013 was 72. 69 per cent had cancer. Sixteen per cent had motor neurone disease. Ninety-three per cent were enrolled in hospice care. So these are not young disabled people being victims of euthanasia, they are dying people, who have access to good services, who decide that they want choice at the end of life. These individuals were also asked what influenced their decisions to ask for assisted dying. Three most cited concerns at end of life were: loss of autonomy (91 per cent); decreasing ability to participate in activities that made life enjoyable (87 per cent); loss of dignity (71 per cent). You could say that all disabled people face these factors. But I think there is a difference to the experience faced by dying people, and the experience of disabled people. The latter group can employ their own personal assistants, participate in society, and not allow their physical limitations to define them. But in my experience of being with friends who are dying, these are not their goals or ambitions. They have had plenty of support from partners and friends. But their activities have been steadily circumscribed, pain has increased, and body functions have been failing. I remember one dear friend, dying of advanced metastatic cancer in her late forties, lying on a hospital bed, doubled up, yellow with jaundice, and in extreme discomfort. I was glad to have the chance to say goodbye, and it was clear to me that none of what I could offer as a disabled activist was at all relevant to her needs at that moment: all she required was loving kindness.

What do disabled people think about assisted dying? In my experience, most disability rights activists are adamantly opposed to the liberalisation of the law. Vocal among them have sometimes been religious people, Catholics like Alison Davis, who was strongly opposed to both abortion and assisted dying.

Inside and outside Parliament, disability rights arguments have been used by religious opponents of the law, and disability activists have lined up next to 'pro-life' banner-wavers.

Yet on this topic, like some others, disability rights leaders seem to be not in tune with the majority of disabled people. Dignity in Dying commissioned a poll from Populus in 2015 which found that 86 per cent of people with a disability supported the Assisted Dying Bill. A similar poll by YouGov in 2013 found that 80 per cent of disabled people supported assisted dying. Similarly, two Australian research studies with people with cancer found the majority supporting assisted dying type proposals. In 2015, I saw one opinion poll published by Disability Rights UK which showed a majority of disabled people opposing assisted suicide. So at worst, it could be concluded that disabled people's views on the subject are mixed. Yet disabled people's organisations have vehemently opposed assisted dying, and the rare individuals such as myself who are prepared to go on record as supporting these legislative proposals are attacked, sometimes on a very personal basis. I think disabled people's organisations should be neutral on assisted dying. They should outline the arguments and evidence on both sides, so that disabled people are empowered to express their own, well-informed, views.

Clearly, there is considerable fear among some activists. But as with some of the fears around hate crime, I believe this is out of proportion. I am not complacent, but I want to believe the best of people. I think that in the medical profession, there is a very strong commitment to keeping people alive. In general, doctors have opposed assisted dying, perhaps because to them it is an admission of defeat, an acceptance that medicine has its limits. Other prominent medical spokespeople, such as (Baroness) Ilora Finlay, have opposed assisted dying, I think because they have a strong commitment to palliative care, and believe that it can always make dying bearable. So I do not fear doctors. I do not think that a few very rare cases such as the murderer Harold Shipman have any implication for the medical profession as a whole, except to reinforce the importance of vigilance.

Similarly, disabled people sometimes fear that family members will wish them speedily dead. They fear that relatives will have one beady eye on their financial resources. They predict that terminally ill people will be pressured to opt for assisted dying. Again, I do not think this is very plausible. I also think that the safeguards in the proposed legislation – having to petition two doctors and one judge – are strong enough to eliminate cases where a dying person is operating under duress. Already, NHS patients have the right to refuse treatment. So if a person is dependent on oxygen or other life support, they can request that this be turned off. Patients can refuse hydration and nutrition, so if they are courageous enough to choose to die from lack of water or food, they can slowly fade away. Yet I have not seen any evidence that any people in these situations are put under pressure to die by family members or doctors.

Opponents also fear the so-called 'slippery slope'. They argue that if you relax the law in the very limited situation of terminal illness, pressure will follow to allow any disabled person access to assisted dying, and following that, to allow any person whatsoever to access assisted dying. But advocates maintain that the vast majority of the population would oppose. No doubt, some euthanasia zealots would still press for further liberalisation, but they would be a tiny minority. Laws are often a compromise – an example is abortion. Some people would favour abortion on demand; others would favour a complete ban. Instead, we have a reasonable measure which sets a limit of viability of 24 weeks, and says only in the most exceptional circumstances can abortion be permitted after this date. This seems a settled position, and it appears very unlikely that abortion law will change at this stage (this does not mean the law is not sometimes abused, which is of course wrong). The fact that a law is a compromise does not mean that it will inevitably slide into permissiveness. At each stage, there is a debate, reasons and evidence are provided, and society and parliament decide. Despite what some more extreme opponents occasionally say, we are not living in a Nazi euthanasia scenario and have no prospect of being there, in a democratic society. We live in a world where there is prejudice, admittedly, but there is also increasing acceptance and support, and considerable sympathy, for disabled people.

But opponents of assisted suicide highlight the risks that this sympathy might generate. For example, if the law was liberalised to allow assisted suicide in the case of terminal illness, people who are living with, for example, tetraplegia, might campaign to be allowed to access assisted suicide. I have witnessed someone who has led a good life, enjoyed considerable success, but now feels that he cannot endure the extreme dependency and limitation of tetraplegia, ask for the right to end his own life. It is very hard not to feel sympathy in a case like this, the same sympathy that we feel for people who are terminally ill. Disability rights activists argue that this benign and supportive feeling is dangerous, because it might lead to a situation where assisted suicide is chosen as the option by many people with impairments who are vulnerable or who cannot access or do not know how to live fulfilled lives with independent living supports.

Opponents of liberalisation also point to welfare benefit changes and reductions in social care expenditure, which have hit disabled people hard. It is true that we seem to be living in an increasingly unsupportive society. People who previously may have received the 24/7 support which they need to lead full lives and participate in society, are now only being given basic support for their self-care needs. This is wrong. Disabled people should not be the main victims of austerity. But I suggest that this campaign for fair welfare and independent living is not so relevant to people who are dying. Sadly, they do not have the prospect of living for many years on inadequate state support. They will qualify for what support exists, because terminally ill people are rightly given accelerated access to Personal Independence Payments and other welfare benefits. If people were making the decision to die early because of a lack of healthcare, hospice care or social support, then this would clearly be a terrible abuse. If the right to assisted suicide was extended beyond people who are terminally ill, this objection would become much more relevant.

In cautiously supporting liberalisation, I would certainly argue in favour of necessary safeguards in law and policy around assisted dying. The law should be restricted to people who are in the terminal stage of terminal illness, for example, people who have six months or less to live, according to reputable medical opinion. People who have depression or mental illness, and are not thinking rationally, should be excluded from coverage. People should have to talk to two doctors and a lawyer or judge, and these professionals should be in unanimity about the suitability of the individual for the assisted dying measure. Safeguards should be in place to ensure that people are free of pressure from relatives, carers, local authorities or service providers. People should have access to all relevant services, whether that is palliative care, including hospice care, independent living and other supports, cancer drugs. In particular, they should have a chance to talk through options and understand how dying can be made easier by medical care. But having complied with all those criteria and considerations, I do think eligible people should be able to choose for themselves.

Assisted dying for terminally ill people hastens an inevitable departure, and completely removes the physical distress and suffering from it. For this reason, I think it is humane and respectful of the personhood of the individual. In a liberal society, law should be protective of vulnerable people, but not paternalistic. I think assisted dying legislation is consistent with disability rights values of having one's voice heard, and having choice and control over one's own life.

CONCLUDING THOUGHTS

Personally, I am very positive about science and medicine, and optimistic about the benefits of our new knowledge and powers. I come from a medical family and have worked closely with geneticists and other clinicians, who in my experience have high integrity and positive values. But I worry about the quality and tone of the debate around genetics and prenatal diagnosis. Too often, arguments are treated as more straightforward than they are. By abstracting from the real world in which people live and choose, issues appear simpler. It is tempting also to see prenatal intervention as either wonderfully progressive and health-improving, or nightmarishly evil and destructive. The truth is far less extreme and more complex.

We need to attend to the complex, messy and irrational world in which people live and make decisions. We need to understand that feelings matter. We should appreciate that choices reflect not medical certainties or consistent logic, but also wider cultural values and beliefs arrangements within a particular society. Above all, we have to ask ourselves an important question: are we willing to welcome and support people with disabilities as future citizens with human rights and a contribution to make to our society? Are we frightened of physical dependency or cognitive limitation? Do we think that life with disability, at any stage of life, can be positive and should be supported?

FURTHER READING

Margaret P. Battin, Agnes van der Heide, Linda Ganzini, Gerrit van der Wal, Bregje D. Onwuteaka-Philipsen. 2007. Legal physician-assisted dying in Oregon and the Netherlands: evidence concerning the impact on patients in 'vulnerable' groups. *Journal of Medical Ethics* 33: 591–597.

Jonathan Glover. 2008. *Choosing Children: genes, disability and design*. Oxford: Oxford University Press.

John Harris. 1992. *Wonderwoman and Superman: the ethics of human biotechnology*. Oxford: Oxford University Press.

Michael Parker. 2012. *Ethical Problems and Genetic Practice*. Cambridge: Cambridge University Press.

Tom Shakespeare. 2014. *Disability Rights and Wrongs Revisited*. London: Routledge.

ADVOCACY AND RESISTANCE

DISABILITY POLITICS

The disabled people's movement has been called 'the last liberation movement': it followed on, and adopted the tactics of, the civil rights movement, women's movement, and lesbian and gay movement that went before. For example, consciousness raising has been a feature of the movement. Whether it was the social model of disability in the UK or the minority rights group model in the United States, activists have taught other disabled people that they did not have to blame themselves or feel bad, they could blame society and feel angry.

In the UK, the Union of the Physically Impaired Against Segregation (UPIAS) were a small group of activists in the 1970s who took a Marxist approach to analysing disabled people's oppression. The Liberation Network of People with Disabilities also discussed oppression, but in a more open and inclusive way, inspired by co-counselling, a personal growth approach. In the 1970s and 1980s, there were many such groups in the UK, out of which emerged the Coalitions of Disabled People in Manchester and Bristol, Leeds and Norfolk, and the Centres for Integrated Living in Hampshire and Greenwich and elsewhere. These local groups began by raising consciousness; they rapidly moved onto campaigning for access and services and equality; finally, they began to be service providers in their own right, providing information and advice and advocacy or independent living support. The largest such groups today have multi-million pound turnovers and contracts with local authorities to provide services to disabled people in their areas.

Direct action has also been a part of the struggle. Activists have campaigned for accessible transport – sometimes by chaining themselves to buses. They have campaigned against patronising images – for example, successfully undermining ITV's charity Telethon. In the United States, a key campaign came after the 1973 Rehabilitation Act, which prohibited discrimination against disabled people in Federal services: activists had to occupy politicians' offices in order to get the new law implemented. By putting their bodies on the line, disability rights activists not only achieved their objectives, they also successfully challenged dominant cultural ideas of disabled people as passive victims.

A key goal of disabled people's movements across the world has been civil rights legislation, first at national level, and finally at global level. For example, in the United States, the Rehabilitation Act was followed by the Education of All Handicapped Children Act (1975), later renamed the Individuals with Disabilities Education Act or IDEA (1990). Because disabled people in the United States were not protected from discrimination by the 1964 Civil Rights Act, there was a continuing campaign for one over-arching piece of legislation. This culminated in the 1990 Americans with Disabilities Act, which set the benchmark for civil rights legislation worldwide.

In the UK, for example, there was a vigorous campaign, bringing together both the radical disability rights activists and the traditional disability charities which resulted in the 1995 Disability Discrimination Act, which was vastly strengthened in 1999 by the Labour government. For example, the Disability Rights Commission replaced the National Disability Council, and gained statutory powers of enforcement; in addition, public bodies were given a statutory duty to promote equality for disabled people. Following a review, all existing equal opportunities legislation, including the Disability Discrimination Act, was brought together in the form of the Equality Act 2010, which includes race, sex, disability, age and other forms of discrimination. While this preserved much of the essence of anti-discrimination, an important dilution was removal of public bodies' requirement to report annually on progress under the disability equality duty. Activists have felt that disability issues have received less support under the unitary Equality and Human Rights Commission than they did under the previous Disability Rights Commission.

The global campaign for civil rights, which brought together peak level bodies such as Disabled People's International, Inclusion International, World Blind Union, World Federation of the Deaf, World Network of Users and Survivors of Psychiatry and others, worked with UN member states for five years to draft the Convention on the Rights of Persons with Disabilities. This global treaty was adopted by the UN in 2006, and came into force in 2008. At the time of writing it has more than 170 ratifications, which means the vast majority of countries in the world have agreed to 'promote, protect and ensure the full and equal enjoyment of all human rights and fundamental freedoms by all persons with disabilities, and to promote respect for their inherent dignity', to quote Article 1. The challenge now is to ensure that all those countries implement the Convention. The process of monitoring compliance falls to the Committee on the Rights of Persons with Disabilities, which meets regularly in Geneva to receive reports from states parties to the Convention, and to interrogate them as to their progress, or lack of it. These public sessions are a way of putting pressure on countries to do more to foster 'progressive realisation' of the human rights of disabled people.

In 2015, the Committee conducted its first investigation into a state which had violated its treaty obligations. That state was the UK, on the grounds of the 'welfare reform' process which had led to cut backs to services and benefits for disabled people. The inquiry concluded that changes to housing benefits and criteria for parts of the Personal Independence Payment, along with a narrowing of social care criteria and the closure of the Independent Living Fund, all 'hindered disabled people's right to live independently and be included in the community'.

Shamefully, after the Committee issued its report about these 'grave human rights violations' in 2016, the Secretary of State for

Work and Pensions, on behalf of the Government, said it 'strongly refuted' the findings and that the Committee held to an 'outdated view of disability which was patronising and offensive'.

DISABILITY ARTS AND CULTURE

From the start, creative work has been part of the advocacy and resistance of the disabled people's movement. Rejecting the occupational therapy approach, where art or craft activities were pastimes which offered an alternative to employment, disability arts has emphasised a political response to oppression. For example, during the 1990s, disability arts cabarets in the UK, with comedians like Barbara Lisicki and Mandy Colleran, and singer-songwriters like Ian Stanton and Johnny Crescendo, helped grow a radical disability rights culture among predominantly disabled audiences. It was here that terms like 'crip' were first recuperated, empowering people and challenging prejudice. From the grass-roots, community arts workshops offered opportunities for disabled people to express themselves as writers, artists and performers. At the same time, non-disabled theatre makers started working with people with learning difficulties. This generated learning difficulty theatre groups in many cities – such as The Lawnmowers in Newcastle and Gateshead, the Blue Teapot Company in Dublin, and Thalia Theatre Company in Norwich. Participation in theatre grew skills and self-confidence and helped promote community living.

The arts activities of the inclusive dance company, Candoco, and the disability theatre company Graeae offered more main-stream options, as they toured ordinary arts venues and demonstrated to mixed audiences that disabled people could make high quality arts work. These companies continue, but now comedians like Laurence Clark and Liz Carr and Francesca Martinez in the UK and Greg Walloch in the United States are also working in mainstream venues, competing with non-disabled comedians on equal terms. Performers such as Mat Fraser push the boundaries in television, theatre and cabaret, while actors such as Peter Dinklage (*Game of Thrones*) and R. J. Mitte (*Breaking Bad*) show that at least a couple of disabled people can get roles in major shows, although the majority of disability roles are still played by non-disabled people. In the visual arts, professionalism has emerged alongside grassroots community arts activities. Yinka Shonibare is one of the generation of Young British Artists, but is not afraid of identifying as a disabled person, while Lucy Jones is a woman with cerebral palsy who does not disavow her impairment, but aims to be judged first and foremost as a painter. From within the disability arts community, Tanya Raabe has painted a series of powerful portraits of disability rights activists. While the disability arts movement is perhaps not as vibrant as it was in the 1990s, organisations such as Shape and websites such as Disability Arts Online still promote the work of the growing numbers of disabled artists.

Partly inspired by disability arts, academics John Swain and Sally French have suggested a new approach to disability, which they term an affirmation model. This combines a focus on the political benefits of identifying with a collectivity, but also a redefinition of the nature of impairment. For example, impairment is seen to bring benefits such as being able to escape role restrictions and social expectations, the possibility of empathy with others and better relationships. In the affirmation approach, disabled people are rejecting dominant values of normality, and asserting the value of life with impairment. For Swain and French, the role of disability culture – for example, disability arts cabarets – is central to this process. An affirmation approach to disability highlights the possibilities of political and cultural resistance, solidarity and meaning making. It rejects the discourses of either tragedy or oppression, and celebrates ordinary everyday life. Yet as the individuals listed above demonstrate, some artists choose to celebrate and explore impairment and disability, whereas others choose to enter the mainstream. Each option offers advantages and both appear valid.

THE DIVERSE CONSTITUENCY

The point has been made already that the disability world is very diverse, and quite possibly people with different impairments do not have much in common. Often, people are thrown together, because they are categorised as disabled or different, and then they have to work out ways of accepting and respecting each other. Strategically, members of different communities have realised that there is strength in numbers, and that they share very similar experiences of exclusion and discrimination.

DEAF COMMUNITY

During the 1970s, Deaf people began organising as a social movement, challenging the idea that they were impaired, and defining themselves increasingly as a linguistic minority, using the model of ethnicity. In this period, slogans such as Deaf Pride and Deaf Power became popular. One of the culminations of this new Deaf identity and political consciousness came with the successful 1988 Deaf President Now protest at Gallaudet University. After the appointment of a hearing President at this university for the Deaf, students exploded into political action, closing down the college in order to demand that the Board of Trustees appoint the first deaf President in the school's history.

The Deaf community have sometimes resisted identification with the mainstream disability movement. Often this is because Deaf people see themselves as a linguistic minority, not as people defined by a medical condition. Of course, some radical disabled people themselves have rejected a medical identity, so perhaps the problem is less one of definition, and more about separate cultures. More of a problem is that dominant disability rights demands – such as inclusive education for all disabled children – are rejected by Deaf communities who want their children separately educated via the medium of Sign Language. Deaf politics found it easier to adopt a straightforward identity politics model, as the movements for Deaf Pride and Deaf Power demonstrate. Social psychologist Henri Tajfel has explored the process of a hitherto excluded community acquiring a 'voice' through social action to enhance the interests of a minority group, which comes to see itself as an oppressed minority. To bolster their self-image, a group exaggerates and values its members' distinctiveness. A sense of injustice and resistance leads to increased identification with the group, which also promotes the self-esteem of its members.

Yet more recently, Deaf politics has got more complex, not least through cochlear implantation. Hearing parents have opted for implants for their children with hearing loss – arguably depriving the Deaf community of more members. However, even adults have now begun to opt for cochlear implants, because technologies promise to help inclusion in a hearing world. Meanwhile, the availability of internet and mobile phone technology means that Deaf people can connect and meet outside the regular Deaf Club setting, whereas in the past, this was the only option to have a social life. Deaf Clubs in many cities are withering as a result. In all these ways, Deafness and hearing loss is becoming a more diverse experience. In developing countries access to sign language and to education is the critical battle, allowing children who have congenital hearing loss, or who have become deafened due to measles or malaria, to gain confidence and qualifications and meet others to campaign for acceptance and inclusion.

MENTAL HEALTH: SURVIVAL AND RECOVERY

In England until into the eighteenth century the approach towards individuals with mental illness was focused on control rather than treatment, with such individuals being confined to Madhouses. One of the earliest examples of service user involvement is the Petition of the Poor Distracted Folk of Bedlam in the 1620s though perhaps the most notable early user group was the Alleged Lunatics' Friend Society created by John Perceval in 1845. In the post-war period, with the use of new drugs such as lithium, a medical model of psychiatry became dominant, with professionals as the experts and service users required merely to comply.

In the early 1970s service users re-emerged as 'survivors' through the growth of organisations such as Campaign Against Psychiatric Oppression and the British Network for Alternatives to Psychiatry. In addition to this other groups such as Survivors Speak Out, UK Advocacy Network (UKAN) and the Hearing Voices Network used the term 'survivor' promoting a positive image of individuals who had survived the mental health services. Such groups were founded to combat a range of issues such as improving conditions of services, closing large long-stay psychiatric hospitals and giving users greater autonomy. During this time, well-known organisations such as Rethink Mental Illness (originally the National Schizophrenia Fellowship) and MIND (1972) also formed.

In the 1980s, Britain saw an increase in mental health service protest with more user groups developing including forums, movements, patient councils and self-help and advocacy groups. It is estimated that the service user movement in the UK has grown from 15 groups in the mid-1980s to over 700 today. Globally, the World Network of Users and Survivors of Psychiatry brings together service user groups, many of whom challenge psychiatric orthodoxies, speaking in terms of difference, not illness.

To take one example: traditionally, auditory and visual hallucinations and delusions have been considered to be symptoms of schizophrenia. Psychiatric treatment – mainly medication – has aimed at removing these symptoms, which are often distressing to people. However, Marius Romme in the Netherlands is a dissident psychiatrist who has, since the late 1980s, taken a less pathologising approach to what he calls 'voice hearing'. Now there are Hearing Voices networks of self-help groups in 29 different countries each of which support people to live better with what are regarded as meaningful differences in perception, reducing participants use of mental health services.

An alternative approach can be found in Japan, where the Bethel House community network hosts an annual 'Hallucination and Delusion Awards' where people with schizophrenia present their delusions and then the audience vote for the delusion of the year. In a similar vein, the British artist Aidan Shingler, in a series of artworks entitled 'Beyond Reason', has taken the thoughts he has had when his schizophrenia is active, and created imagery which communicates to others what these experiences are like.

While some survivors avoid mental health services and seek other forms of support, the recovery movement has influenced mainstream provision. Recovery Colleges are an innovation in many mental health trusts, where an educational approach, based on co-production, seeks to help people affected by mental illness lead better lives. This includes employing peer support workers – people who themselves have experienced mental illness – to work alongside patients as role models and psychological supporters, emphasising hope and social inclusion.

LEARNING DIFFICULTIES: SELF-ADVOCACY

The self-advocacy movement offers people with learning difficulties a place where they can meet friends, feel affirmed, and
celebrate their lives. Part of this is challenging stereotypes of
'feeble-mindedness' or 'idiocy' and re-affirming dignity and the
right to speak out for oneself. Opposition to labelling is very
strong amongst self-advocates, who wish to be treated as individuals, not to be defined in terms of what is wrong with them.
Working together with non-disabled supporters or with family
members, or with researchers, people with learning difficulties
have told their stories, campaigned for better provision, and
created spaces where they can be together and be valued.

At the local level, self-advocacy groups meet to support people
living in the community. Whereas in the past, it was organisations
'for' people, such as Mencap, now increasingly it is organisations
'of' people, such as Opening Doors or Speak Up or similar
groups that represents the voice of people with learning difficulties. Performing arts groups such as The Lawnmowers in
Gateshead or Blue Teapot Theatre Company in Dublin or Thalia
Theatre Company in Norwich make work that speaks directly to
other people with learning difficulties, but also demonstrates to a
non-disabled audience what can be achieved.

In the past, the only option for people with learning
difficulties was a day centre, or more likely a residential
institution. Now, arts organisations, social firms and other enterprises offer alternative ways of life. Much of this is non-disabled
people living and working alongside people with learning difficulties. For example, the L'Arche movement was founded by
Canadian Jean Vanier, and follows Christian principles in enabling
people with learning difficulties to live in the community in
shared houses with non-disabled supporters. There are now 143
communities in 35 countries worldwide, supporting 3,500
people in living or working together with non-disabled people.

At the national level, organisations like People First have
offered an authentic voice of people with learning difficulties. In
the United States, Arc developed out of the former Association
of Retarded Citizens and offers a similar campaigning and advocacy voice. At the international level, Inclusion International

campaigned for the Convention on the Rights of Persons with Disabilities, and has since published guides to interpreting and implementing it in the learning difficulties field. Inclusion International now comprises 200 member confederations in 115 countries worldwide, supporting people with learning difficulties and their families.

AUTISM AND NEURO-DIVERSITY

Over the last few decades, many families and individuals have been affected by autism. Whether this is because the condition is more common, or whether other forms of learning difficulty have been relabelled as autism spectrum conditions, is unclear. Prevalence of autism is thought to be around 1 per cent. Researchers suggest that approximately half of people with autism spectrum conditions also have learning difficulties. Families have found the onset of autism to be distressing, and have striven to find therapies to alleviate symptoms or change behaviours. Sometimes rather extreme dietary or sensory or behavioural modification regimes have been suggested.

Meanwhile, the neurodiversity movement challenges the idea that autism spectrum conditions are problems and instead try to validate people whose brains may work in different ways. This often includes other neurological conditions such as Tourette's and ADHD. Neurodiversity advocates such as Arie Ne'eman in the United States speak out for an acceptance of the diversity of human experience and functioning. The focus is on accommodation and inclusion, not prevention and cure. As with other disability rights arguments, the obligation is for society to change, rather than individuals to be cured. This argument has been put most forcefully by the journalist Steve Silberman in his award-winning book *Neurotribes*, which tells the story of autism research and explores raised awareness of autism and the need for acceptance of neurodiversity.

After all, many people on the autism spectrum make major contributions, from the quantum mechanics pioneer Paul Dirac, who many people think was probably on the spectrum, to many of the so-called geeks in Silicon Valley who developed the internet, ICT and social media that everyone else relies on. Writers such as the animal behaviourist Temple Grandin and Australian musician Donna Williams have written memoirs and other books which have challenged the neurotypical world to accept their different approaches to thinking and relating. For example, the architectural artist Stephen Wiltshire is another 'savant', who is skilled in the creation of astonishingly detailed drawings of buildings and cityscapes, even after only a very brief look. Wiltshire now has a successful artistic career, and has been the recipient of awards including an MBE.

However, not all autistic people are geeks or savants. Naturally, the advocates for neurodiversity tend to be the less affected and more communicative of those people affected. Many families are struggling to support their learning disabled children with autism, particularly as they transition from paediatric to adult services. Approximately a quarter of these young people will never develop verbal skills. The new stereotype of exceptional eccentric does not account for the many children with profound learning difficulties and often challenging behaviour, or the increased risk that people on the autistic spectrum end up in the criminal justice system because of inappropriate or aggressive behaviours. Above all, as Silberman stresses, autistic spectrum conditions cover a wide range, and many different abilities and traits.

ALLIES

While non-disabled people do not have direct personal experience of impairment and disability, they can experience disability indirectly. For example, many prominent disability researchers – including Lennard Davis in the United States or Rannveig Traustadóttir in Iceland – are themselves children of Deaf or disabled parents. Others are siblings or parents of disabled people, for example the UK autism researcher Lorna Wing, or even partners of disabled people. Whether as researchers, advocates or policymakers, these individuals do bring a personal understanding of the complexity of disabled lives, and a commitment to making them better. They may have experienced prejudice and discrimination themselves, because of their associations with disabled people. Moreover, non-disabled people can become disabled –

and often do, as a result of ageing. Although everyone has a stake in disability policies and politics, some people have a more direct lived experience and viewpoint, which should be prioritised in policy and practice.

INTERSECTIONALITY

As well as differences between the impairment groups, within each group there are differences based on class, gender, ethnicity and sexuality. The experience of a health condition will differ – for example, a family with a child with Down syndrome may have a much harder time if they lack material resources and cultural capital, or face racism within their neighbourhood. Often disadvantage intersects, as with gender and disability. Sometimes, an aspect of someone's identity may be overshadowed, such as sexuality. Or conversely, someone might channel their feelings of difference into their sexuality, and ignore their disability.

GENDER AND SEXUALITY

More boys than girls have impairments, and men have traditionally been more likely to do the activities that result in traumatic injuries. But in older age, there are more disabled women than men, and overall, more women than men are disabled. Different conditions are also gendered: MS, for example, is two to three times more common in women than men. Conversely, there are more males than females with autism. There are twice as many women than men with depression, although overall rates of mental illness are almost the same for men and women. But approximately three-quarters of people who commit suicide are male.

Stereotypes of masculinity and disability seem in conflict (how can you be a man if you lack physical power?), whereas femininity and disability could be seen as reinforcing discourses of dependency and passivity. In practice, disabled men might assert their physicality through wheelchair sports – or may redefine masculinity in creative ways. Disabled women may find themselves liberated from stereotypical femininity. This may come at a cost, if they are then considered to be asexual as well.

As with other areas of domestic labour, women bear the brunt of informal care responsibility. Whether it is mothers looking after disabled children, or daughters looking after older disabled relatives, care can be experienced as burdensome, particularly if families are under-supported by the state. Only in older age do men do an equivalent share of care to women, because older husbands may often find themselves carers for wives with illnesses or impairments. Perhaps for these reasons, feminism seems to have taken more account of disability than left-wing politics. There's a shared emphasis, also, in the idea of the personal being political.

Traditionally, disabled people have been regarded as asexual. In practice, throughout the world, many disabled people have partners, and some have children. Others are lesbian, gay, bisexual or transgender. In Britain, the voluntary group Regard has been a haven for LGBT disabled people for several decades, campaigning for access and recognition with the gay community, but also for support and inclusion in the mainstream world. For example, there is growing evidence that LGBT people in the social care system or LGBT people with learning difficulties can face ignorance or prejudice from personal assistants and care workers, not to mention family members. The late pop star George Michael was a great supporter of self-organised disabled groups like Regard and many others, channelling thousands of pounds anonymously through the Platinum Trust.

DISABILITY AND ETHNICITY

Black and minority ethnic disabled people may face prejudice within families and communities on the basis of disability – and racism from health or social care providers. More even than other disabled people, black and minority ethnic disabled people may face low expectations of their potential, and end up with poor self-confidence. People of African and Afro-Caribbean origins are disproportionately represented in mental health services, due largely to the experience of living in a racist society. There may be an assumption that Asian families 'look after their own' and do not require services. Religious and cultural identities may not be catered for within services. People may 'fall between' disability services or organisations, and those for minority ethnic communities. People may be ignorant of the services that are available to them. Because of racism and ignorance, black and minority ethnic disabled people and families often request specialist services, according to research conducted for the Joseph Rowntree Foundation. For example, the Asian People with Disabilities Alliance works in the UK and also in South Asia to provide services and challenge prejudice. In the United States, the National Black Disability Coalition has advocated for disabled people of colour since 1990.

DISABILITY STUDIES

This chapter has discussed disability politics and disability culture. But another radical arena has been disability studies. Here, sociologists, historians, cultural studies researchers and others have approached their subjects with a new lens and different priorities. To take just a few examples:

- Colin Barnes conducted sociological research with disabled people and staff in a day centre;
- Jenny Morris interviewed women with disabilities;
- with my colleagues Kath Gillespie-Sells and Dominic Davies I talked to disabled people about sexuality and relationships;
- Paul Longmore and Anne Borsay pioneered disability history;
- Rosemarie Garland-Thomson developed a cultural analysis of staring; and
- Lennard Davis traced the emergence of the category of normality.

These and hundreds of other researchers have asked different questions and studied those normally hidden from history or society, while committed to the emancipation of disabled people. Disability studies has emulated lesbian and gay or queer studies, or post-colonial studies or women's studies, in challenging both society and the academy itself to change.

It's impossible to give more than a flavour of this research. In the UK, it might be helpful to think of three waves of disability studies. The first way is represented by Michael Oliver, whose book *The Politics of Disablement* (1990) was path-breaking in establishing a new sociological field. Meanwhile Vic Finkelstein never produced a unified theory, but he did generate dozens of provocations, exploring the social model of disability, looking at disability at different phases of history, exploring the helped-helper relationship. He also created an Open University module on The Disabling Society, which was the first academic course taking a disability studies approach. Jenny Morris, in a series of pioneering books such as *Pride Against Prejudice* (1991), took a more feminist perspective on disability, highlighted the role of culture and attitudes, and conducted detailed research on independent living and social policy. Colin Barnes founded a very influential MA in Disability Studies at Leeds University, and supported many disabled people to enter research. Len Barton's major contribution, aside from his own important work on inclusive education, was to establish and edit the journal *Disability and Society*.

The second wave is represented by scholars such as Alan Roulstone, Mark Priestley, Carol Thomas, Nicholas Watson and myself, all of whom have worked in the mainstream of sociology or social policy. Some of these researchers took a more critical perspective on the social model; others drew on theory from feminism or other areas of social science to explore how disabling factors operated, or how disability was lived. Meanwhile, topics such as health and employment were investigated in greater detail, as disability studies became a more established academic discipline. Finally, the third wave came with scholars such as David Bolt, Dan Goodley, Dan Grech, Hannah Morgan who represent an explosion of interest in theory, culture, identity and difference.

Another way of looking at disability studies would be to distinguish *materialist* disability studies, influenced by Marxism and centred on the traditional social model (Oliver, Barnes, Finkelstein, Barton) from *critical realist* disability studies, seeing disability as an interaction between a person with a health condition and wider contexts (Watson, Anders Gustavsson, myself) and *critical disability studies* (Goodley, Davis, Helen Meekosha), which pays more attention to the construction of categories and the role of culture. In general, this latter approach is more represented in North

America, with scholars such as Rosemarie Garland-Thomson, Lennard Davis, David Mitchell, Sharon Snyder, Rob McRuer, most of whom have training in literary studies, not social science, and sometimes have a different approach to evidence.

Disability studies has become very popular with students and researchers, because it is new and radical and there are so many questions to be asked and answered. In the United States, the Society for Disability Studies, founded in 1986 by pioneering disabled sociologist Irving Zola and others, has been meeting annually for many years. The Disability Studies Association in the UK has been meeting bi-annually since 2003, alternating with the Nordic Network of Disability Research, which will hold its fourteenth conference in 2017. Disability studies has spread outside the English-speaking world: a new European conference has begun meeting, hosted by the European journal *Alter*. Other networks have sprung up, for example, in Canada, France, Italy and the Netherlands.

Despite this growth over recent decades, disability studies has also faced challenges. For example, should the emphasis be on creating a new discipline within the academy through high quality scholarship and the development of undergraduate and postgraduate programmes, or on contributing to disability politics, through engaged and emancipatory research? Is it better to foster a separate discipline, or to ensure that disability is researched within existing disciplines? What is the place of non-disabled scholars? How should a balance be achieved between social and political research and research in cultural or literary studies? Is there a danger of too much abstract theory and not enough empirical research? None of these questions threatens the core values of the discipline, but they all need to be considered.

NOTHING ABOUT US WITHOUT US

A central theme in this chapter, and indeed this whole book, is the principle of user involvement. Rather than non-disabled people deciding for disabled people, disabled people should, wherever possible, decide for themselves. In some countries, such as Uganda, this has meant places being reserved for disabled people at all levels of the political system. I was impressed, when

I did research with successful disabled people in Kampala, to hear from many of them that their ambition was to enter politics, or even become president. In Britain, fewer disabled people have become politicians – although Anne Begg and David Blunkett offer good precedents as members of the House of Commons. Blunkett has now joined other disabled people such as Jane Campbell and Tanni Grey-Thompson in the House of Lords. Generally, due to the older age profile, there are more disabled people in the House of Lords, even though they don't always identify with the values of the disability movement.

User involvement also explains why disabled people have started their own organisations and networks, rather than relied on the traditional unrepresentative charitable organisations. User involvement is also an important principle in social services and other local government provision: hearing from the people directly affected, through the principle of co-production of services, should mean that social care and recovery services are more appropriate and effective. Rather than experts determining what is best for people, people should use their own lived experience to determine the shape of provision. This is the principle of 'expertise by experience', which accords closely with the key disability movement slogan of 'nothing about us without us'. The corollary of experts by experience is that professionals should be 'on tap but not on top'. It is certainly the case that specialist expertise – for example, from lawyers and economists and doctors and educationalists – is required. But this should not mean that professionals have all the power, and disabled people have none. I remember how social work academic David Brandon quoted Tolstoy:

> I sit on a man's back choking him and making him carry me, and yet assure myself and others that I am sorry for him and wish to lighten his load by all means possible ... except by getting off his back.

User involvement, or coproduction, is also important in the area of research. The principle of *emancipatory research* was developed by Michael Oliver and others in the 1990s, to highlight the importance of adopting a social model approach, of having a commitment to social change, and of working closely with disabled people's organisations. Researchers on learning difficulty have led the way in co-production of research, genuinely including people with lived experience as advisors, and even as researchers. The idea is that the process of doing research, not just the results of doing research, should be empowering to participants and beneficiaries. Major independent grant givers, such as the Rowntree Foundation and the Big Lottery Fund have made user involvement a condition of funding schemes. These approaches have been widely influential. The National Institute for Health Research (NIHR), the research arm of the NHS, now mandates 'patient and public involvement' in research projects, including basic clinical research. As a result, disability researchers who are themselves disabled – or Deaf, or with experience of mental health conditions – have grown in number and influence. However, the lower numbers of disabled people going into higher education limits growth in the number of disabled scholars.

CONCLUSION

The UK disability movement exemplifies both the strengths and the weaknesses of identity politics. Social psychologist Henri Tajfel has explored the process of a hitherto excluded community acquiring a 'voice' through social action to enhance the interests of a minority group, which comes to see itself as an oppressed minority. To bolster their self-image, a group exaggerates and values its members' distinctiveness. A sense of injustice and resistance leads to increased identification with the group, which also promotes the self-esteem of its members. While the movement has inspired many disabled people and achieved key goals such as civil rights legislation and improvements to access and attitudes, it has also occasionally been riven by ideological and personality disputes.

As local organisations have become service providers, and as funding for campaigning groups has dried up, it has become more difficult for disabled people in Britain to speak with one voice. Also, energies were united in campaigning for anti-discrimination legislation: when this was achieved in 1995, and strengthened in following years, the impetus for radicalism died away. Today, many disabled people do not identify as disabled, and only a minority have heard of the social model of disability, let alone espouse it. However, many grassroots support groups and advocacy organisations do thrive and survive. Younger disabled people to some extent have taken the victories of disability rights for granted, just as younger women may not identify so strongly with feminism. Now, as these gains are under attack in a period of austerity, new generations of disabled people may become radicalised.

Political theorist Nancy Fraser talks about social movements having twin goals of redistribution (i.e. improving material conditions) and recognition (i.e. validating different forms of life). This applies well to the disability movements and self-advocacy groups described in this chapter in developing countries as well as developed countries. However, Fraser also diagnoses how identity politics can become inward looking and sectarian. She points out that the diversity of experiences and affiliations can become suppressed in terms of a shared ideology and identity. Fraser suggests that the goal of trying to assert the value of a group is misplaced. Instead, the aim should be to assert the equal status of individuals, what she calls identitarian, rather than identity politics, focusing on parity of esteem.

Meanwhile, the UN Convention on the Rights of Persons with Disabilities may also be more limited in impact than its proposers would have hoped. While most countries in the world have ratified the treaty, actual progress towards implementing disability rights has been slower than hoped. The Convention offers a standard for states to try and attain, but it lacks teeth and ultimately relies on voluntary good practice by states and other human rights duty bearers. The recent UK experience shows that some governments will simply ignore the recommendations of the Committee on the Rights of Persons with Disabilities. Nor does the Convention encompass all dimensions of disability. Families, for example, are largely left out, and there is only the briefest mention of indigenous people with disabilities, who face particular struggles in Canada, Australia, New Zealand and Latin America, and who may understand impairment and disability in very different ways to the majority culture.

There's a lot still for disability activists to be angry about. In the UK, austerity seems to have impacted disabled people disproportionately, rolling back some of the advances that had been made in the previous twenty years. There is growing attention to the higher likelihood that disabled people, particularly people with learning difficulties, will become victims of violence. There are health inequalities, particularly for people with learning difficulties or mental health conditions, which mean that people die earlier than they should. Globally, disabled children are disproportionately likely to be excluded from a good education. Everywhere, it's difficult for disabled people to access transport and get around like other people. Attitudes are still unreformed, for example around sex and relationships. So the campaigns will continue.

Two messages should be reinforced. First, disability is not about victimhood or even oppression. It is about survival and resistance and recovery. Joining together, campaigning for inclusion, disabled people in greater numbers than ever before are changing the world and removing barriers. Second, disability is very diverse, perhaps even more diverse than other equalities issues. Think of the thousands of health conditions, intersecting with the other forms of diversity, in the many different contexts in which people live and work and make meaning. There is rarely one problem or one explanation or one solution that applies for everyone. People understand themselves and affiliate in different ways, and this may change as their lives continue. It seems to me that openness to these possibilities – to letting a thousand flowers bloom – is the only way forward.

FURTHER READING

Jane Campbell and Michael Oliver. 1995. *Disability Politics: understanding our past, changing our future*. London: Routledge.

James Charlton. 2000. *Nothing About Us Without Us: disability oppression and empowerment*. Berkeley, CA: University of California Press.

Lennard Davis. 2013. *The Disability Studies Reader*. New York: Routledge.

Nancy Fraser. 2010. *Scales of Justice: reimagining political space in a globalizing world*. New York: Columbia University Press.

Tom Shakespeare. 2015. *Disability Research Today: international perspectives*. Abingdon: Routledge.

Roddy Slorach. 2016. *A Very Capitalist Condition: a history and politics of disability*. London: Bookmarks.

APPENDIX

DIALOGUE ON PRENATAL SCREENING

I first wrote this text in 2000. With minor tweaks, it seems to remain relevant today, as a guide through some of the complexities of debates on prenatal screening. Anne is an opponent of prenatal screening, while John is an advocate of prenatal screening.

ANNE: Genetics is just the same as eugenics. It's about eliminating 'lives unworthy of life', which is what the Nazis did.

JOHN: I assume you're not implying that geneticists are Nazis, because that's untrue and offensive. But when it comes to eugenics, it depends what you mean by the word: it is notoriously difficult to agree a definition. The main differences between early twentieth century eugenics and the present practice of prenatal screening are that pre-1945 it was a matter of state policy, and it often involved coercion. In present-day Western countries, pregnancy termination is the free choice of individual women and men, within the parameters of the law.

ANNE: Well, I'm not opposing a woman's right to choose. If a woman decides not to continue with her pregnancy, then that's up to her. But choosing whether or not to be pregnant is a different choice from deciding which fetus to be pregnant with. I support that first right to choose, but not the second. I think it is discriminatory to make that choice on the basis of the characteristics of the fetus.

JOHN: I'm not sure you can separate the issues of 'being pregnant' and 'being pregnant with a particular fetus'. Consider the hypothetical case of an unmarried sixteen-year-old girl who becomes pregnant. Her decision as to whether to continue and become a single parent might be different in the case of a potentially non-disabled baby than it would be in the case of a potentially affected baby. She might decide she could cope with the former situation – knowing that day care and all sorts of other support might be available – but that she could not cope being the single parent of a baby who had high support and care needs. And surely it is counter-intuitive to allow women to exercise their right to choose termination for social reasons – such as failed contraception, or a change of heart, or being too old or young, or having too many children – but to deny it in the cases of diagnosed serious fetal impairment?

ANNE: Okay, I allow your point that choice is an important principle. But I don't believe that women and men are exercising free and non-constrained choices in practice, for several reasons. First, they are not given full information. Sometimes they are not given proper clinical information about the particular impairment that has been diagnosed. Usually they are not given full social information on what it's like to have that impairment, and the quality-of-life implications. They are rarely told about the psychological impacts of termination of pregnancy. And they are never provided with the perspectives of disabled people themselves, who are the real experts on being disabled. Second, doctors and other professionals are biased against disabled people. They are ignorant about disability. They think disability is a tragedy to be avoided at all costs. They do not counsel non-directively. They believe screening is a good thing, and this influences their patients. Third, the clinical context influences the choices made: for example, making a test available implies the desirability of that test. Antenatal testing is like a conveyor belt, and many women are not given the time and information to make an informed decision. Finally, society is increasingly blaming women for not having tests or not having terminations. For all these reasons, there is no real choice at the moment, and women are not supported to continue with pregnancy, if they want to do so.

JOHN: I accept your argument. Choice at the moment is rather limited. Society needs to ensure that resources are invested to enable women and men to make fully informed choices. But, if we managed to achieve that, then you would have no reason to prevent women having the choice of terminating pregnancy affected by impairment, if they wanted to, would you?

ANNE: I'm not sure. I don't like the idea of people trying to avoid the birth of disabled people. It's like saying disabled people aren't worthy of life …

JOHN: That's not necessarily the case. I can think of four reasons a woman might choose to avoid the birth of a disabled child. One is because they don't think disabled people should exist, or because they think that disabled people aren't worthy of life. Another is the argument that society should not have to pay the costs of supporting disabled people. These both seem to me to be morally dangerous. I would join you in opposing them, and I would call them 'eugenic' reasons. But the second two reasons seem to me to be important. One is that impairment involves suffering and physical difficulties, and it is unfair to bring people into the world to suffer. The second is that it is often difficult for the parents and siblings of disabled children. There is sometimes a very negative impact on the whole family. Relationships break up, and brothers and sisters may become neglected or resentful.

ANNE: I am glad you agree that your first two reasons are oppressive and should be opposed. But I think you've missed the point about disability. Both your second two reasons are not really about what it's like to have an impairment. They are about the way society treats someone with impairment. Disabled people say their real problems are discrimination and prejudice in society. That's what makes life difficult for disabled people and their families. We should remove the social factors that cause suffering and isolation, rather than remove disabled people from the world. We need social engineering, not genetic engineering!

JOHN: Okay, fair enough, I agree we should try and change the world, although I reckon that it might be much harder than you think to change some of these social problems. But surely, not all impairments are the same. There are some impairments which are invariably very difficult. Babies die in their first year of life, or people die before their twentieth birthday, or people live very difficult lives with limited consciousness and self-awareness, or else with extreme pain and physical difficulties. However much you change society, surely these problems will remain and should be avoided if possible?

ANNE: Well that's just it. I don't think it's up to us to try and remove impairments from the world. Impairment is a fact of life – after all, we're all going to die. Being alive involves suffering. We shouldn't be playing at God.

JOHN: Well, impairment may be inevitable, but that doesn't mean we don't have a duty to try and minimise it, especially when it is very severe and debilitating. After all, we agree on some tactics for removing impairment, such as the vaccination of children, or mine clearance, or looking both ways when we cross the road. Nobody would have a problem with impairment prevention, would they?

ANNE: I think there's a difference between impairment prevention and removing people with impairment from the world. And where do you draw the line? If you are giving women the right to choose, does that mean the right to terminate pregnancy on the basis of the sex of the potential child, or perhaps sexuality or intelligence? If you are going to be consistent about choice, then why stop at impairment?

JOHN: There is no requirement to be either totally pro-choice, or totally anti-choice. Termination of pregnancy is a morally significant act. It involves halting life once it has started, and should not be entered into lightly. Because termination of pregnancy is morally significant and important, it should be chosen only when the alternative would be much worse for the parents or potential child. For this reason, termination of pregnancy on grounds of personality characteristics – for example, gender and sexuality – should be avoided.

ANNE: It's all very well resorting to philosophical arguments. But the fact is, that I might not have been born, if these selective termination techniques had been available to my parents' generation …

JOHN: Your statement has immense emotional weight, but it does not make sense. Saying 'I would not have been born' is not logical. The point is that you were born. Prior to your birth, there was no 'I'. Only after your birth was there an 'I'. Souls do not wait in limbo before birth, being prevented from coming into the world by particular acts of contraception or termination of pregnancy.

ANNE: Okay, I accept that, if you want to be pedantic. What I meant was, these techniques stop disabled people in general from being born.

JOHN: But that's not strictly true either. You have accepted that termination of pregnancy is morally acceptable, presumably on the basis that up to a certain stage of pregnancy – say 24 weeks – there is no 'person' involved, just a 'potential person'. Termination of pregnancy stops a collection of cells developing further. It does not stop a disabled person being born. However, the effect of selective termination may be to reduce the number of disabled people in the world.

ANNE: That's exactly what I mean. Selective termination reduces diversity. And what's more, terminating fetuses affected by the same condition as me is a form of discrimination against disabled people. It's a judgement on me and on my life. It will lead to more prejudice against disabled people.

JOHN: I am not sure that there is any evidence that selective termination of pregnancy increases prejudice against disabled people. In China, for example, there is a strong eugenic policy, but there is also increasingly good provision for disabled people. And the fact that we take a sugar lump inoculation against polio does not cause discrimination against people with polio. Prevention and support are not incompatible.

Again, I can see the emotional relevance of your feeling discriminated against because of a screening programme designed to eliminate your impairment, but I don't think it is just or rational. After all, let's say you got your way, and out of respect to you, society decided to prohibit selective termination on the basis of your impairment. What would you say, in twenty years' time, to the person who was born with the impairment, when they complain that you stopped the technology being used to prevent the birth of people with that impairment? Why should they suffer because the idea of impairment prevention makes you unhappy or feel discriminated against?

ANNE: Okay, maybe I shouldn't have talked about discrimination. But I notice that you haven't dealt with my argument about diversity. I still think that selective screening could go too far. I accept that people should have reproductive choice, but I don't want to see a world in which all impairment has been eliminated. We should value every individual, and we should support difference. I want to see these technologies carefully regulated, I want to see informed and supported choices, and I think we should recognise the contribution which disabled people make to the world, and their right to be a part of it. If we challenge the prejudice and fear which surrounds disability, prospective parents would be less likely to feel that termination was the only answer.

JOHN: I don't have any problem agreeing with that. I can see why you feel insulted and denigrated by the rhetoric which supporters of genetic intervention sometimes adopt. I think we should be careful not to say disability is invariably a tragedy, and I think we should try and reduce the discrimination which often makes the lives of disabled people so much more difficult. But I do believe that we should offer women and men access to screening information, and give them a free choice about whether to continue with pregnancy.

Perhaps there's also a difference between testing, which involves families who already have a history of genetic conditions, and who know what they involve, and screening, which extends genetic intervention to the whole population. Screening is often introduced on the basis of cost-benefit calculations about avoiding the birth of disabled people. It seems to be where genetics comes uncomfortably close to eugenics. Perhaps we should be in less of a hurry to introduce the latest tests, or extend them as widely as possible to knowing the whole genome. Biotech corporations might be keen for us to take advantage of these technologies, but if we cannot guarantee that people will be informed and supported to make the best choices, then perhaps it is too risky to push onwards with this type of screening.

GLOSSARY

ASSISTIVE DEVICES Technologies such as wheelchairs, hearing aids, communication devices to improve functioning of disabled people.

ASSISTED DYING When a person who is terminally ill receives help to end their own life without pain; also known as *physician-assisted suicide.*

COMMUNITY-BASED REHABILITATION (CBR) Found particularly in developing countries, a strategy for promoting inclusion of disabled people in education, health, livelihood and social activities through community workers and community projects.

DEAF With a capital D, refers to people with hearing loss who use Sign language to communicate.

DISABILITY Narrowly, the outcome of the interaction between a person with impairment and the wider physical and social context; broadly, used variously to refer to both the impairment, and the functional deficit, and the social experience.

EUGENICS A word coined by Francis Galton in 1883 to refer to 'the science of the improvement of the human germ plasm though better breeding'; now usually refers to coercive policies of population improvement through sterilisation or genetic testing and termination of pregnancy.

EUTHANASIA Intentionally ending a life, to relieve suffering; often refers to the involuntary extermination programmes of the Nazi regime.

FALSE NEGATIVE When a screening test says the pregnancy is free of a condition, when in reality it is affected.

FALSE POSITIVE When a screening test says the pregnancy is affected by a condition, when in reality it is not.

'FEEBLE-MINDED' Out-dated term for *learning difficulty* or *intellectual disability*.

IMPAIRMENT A problem in body function or structure experienced by an individual (such as loss of a limb or a sense, or paralysis).

INCIDENCE The number of new cases of a health condition in a time period.

INCLUSION Where pupils with special needs spend most or all of their time with non-special needs pupils in mainstream schools.

INSTITUTIONALISATION A policy of children or adults with disabilities living in residential institutions, rather than the community.

INTEGRATION Where pupils with special needs are educated in special classrooms within mainstream schools.

INTELLECTUAL DISABILITY The international term for *intellectual impairment* or *learning disability*.

LEARNING DIFFICULTY The term for *intellectual impairment* which is preferred by people who experience it themselves.

LEARNING DISABILITY Term for *intellectual impairment* used, for example, in the NHS.

LESS ELIGIBILITY In social policy, making welfare benefits

inadequate or undesirable so people would rather work than claim them.

PRE-IMPLANTATION GENETIC DIAGNOSIS (PGD) A technique used by families affected by inherited genetic conditions: embryos are created through IVF, then tested at a very early stage to see if they are affected by a condition; embryos free of the condition can then be implanted in the mother's womb.

PREVALENCE The number of cases of a health condition in a population.

REASONABLE ADJUSTMENT Also called *reasonable accommodation* (US); refers to assistance or changes in the workplace that will enable a disabled employee to do his or her job.

RECOVERY In mental health, the belief that it is possible for someone to regain a meaningful life, despite serious mental illness.

REHABILITATION THERAPIES Clinical approaches such as physiotherapy, occupational therapy, speech and language therapy, rehabilitation counselling which help restore or maintain functioning.

RESTRICTED GROWTH Also known as *dwarfism* or *short stature*; may result from one of 200 different genetic or developmental conditions.

SELF-ADVOCACY People with learning difficulties speaking for themselves, or more widely, the civil rights movement of people with learning difficulties.

SENSITIVITY In screening, the ability of a test to identify true cases of a condition.

SOCIAL MODEL The idea that people with impairments are disabled by society, not by their bodies.

SPECIAL EDUCATION Specially designed teaching to meet the unique needs of a child with a disability; can be delivered in either a mainstream or segregated setting.

SPECIAL SCHOOL Where children with disabilities receive special education in a segregated setting.

SPECIFIC LEARNING DISABILITIES Conditions such as dyslexia and dyspraxia which affect a child's ability to learn, but where intellect is not impaired.

SPECIFICITY In screening, the ability of a test to avoid false positives.

STERILISATION Treatment to make it impossible for a person to reproduce, for example vasectomy or tubal ligation.

INDEX

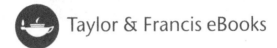 Taylor & Francis eBooks

---

Helping you to choose the right eBooks for your Library

Add Routledge titles to your library's digital collection today. Taylor and Francis ebooks contains over 50,000 titles in the Humanities, Social Sciences, Behavioural Sciences, Built Environment and Law.

Choose from a range of subject packages or create your own!

Benefits for you

» Free MARC records
» COUNTER-compliant usage statistics
» Flexible purchase and pricing options
» All titles DRM-free.

REQUEST YOUR FREE INSTITUTIONAL TRIAL TODAY

Free Trials Available
We offer free trials to qualifying academic, corporate and government customers.

Benefits for your user

» Off-site, anytime access via Athens or referring URL
» Print or copy pages or chapters
» Full content search
» Bookmark, highlight and annotate text
» Access to thousands of pages of quality research at the click of a button.

eCollections – Choose from over 30 subject eCollections, including:

Archaeology	Language Learning
Architecture	Law
Asian Studies	Literature
Business & Management	Media & Communication
Classical Studies	Middle East Studies
Construction	Music
Creative & Media Arts	Philosophy
Criminology & Criminal Justice	Planning
Economics	Politics
Education	Psychology & Mental Health
Energy	Religion
Engineering	Security
English Language & Linguistics	Social Work
Environment & Sustainability	Sociology
Geography	Sport
Health Studies	Theatre & Performance
History	Tourism, Hospitality & Events

For more information, pricing enquiries or to order a free trial, please contact your local sales team:
www.tandfebooks.com/page/sales

 Routledge
Taylor & Francis Group

The home of
Routledge books

www.tandfebooks.com

9 781138 651395